Connie W. Bales is Associate Director of the Sarah W. Stedman Center for Nutritional Studies, Associate Professor of Medicine, and Senior Fellow at the Center for the Study of Aging and Human Development at Duke University Medical Center. She holds a doctorate in Nutrition Science and is also a Registered Dietitian.

Steve J. Schwab is Professor of Medicine and Clinical Director of the Division of Nephrology at Duke University Medical Center. He serves on the editorial boards of Kidney International, The American Journal of Kidney Diseases, and Advances in Renal Replacement Therapy. He is actively involved in research dealing with dialysis, end-stage renal disease, and chronic renal failure.

Dorothy W. Bartholomay is a Registered Dietitian with a master's degree in public health who specializes in the dietary treatment of kidney disease. She is the Clinic Dietitian at Duke University's Dialysis Center and is involved in research into various aspects of nephrology.

Dietary Approaches to Healthy Living
from
The Sarah W. Stedman Center
for Nutritional Studies at
Duke University Medical Center

Eating Well, Living Well with Diabetes
Eating Well, Living Well with Hypertension
Eating Well, Living Well with Osteoporosis

EATING WELL, LIVING WELL
with
KIDNEY DISEASE

Steve J. Schwab, M.D.
Dorothy W. Bartholomay, M.P.H., R.D.

Connie W. Bales, PH.D., R.D.
Series Editor

with Michelle McGee

VIKING

VIKING
Published by the Penguin Group
Penguin Books USA Inc., 375 Hudson Street,
New York, New York 10014, U.S.A.
Penguin Books Ltd, 27 Wrights Lane,
London W8 5TZ, England
Penguin Books Australia Ltd, Ringwood,
Victoria, Australia
Penguin Books Canada Ltd, 10 Alcorn Avenue,
Toronto, Ontario, Canada M4V 3B2
Penguin Books (N.Z.) Ltd, 182–190 Wairau Road,
Auckland 10, New Zealand

Penguin Books Ltd, Registered Offices:
Harmondsworth, Middlesex, England

First published in 1997 by Viking Penguin,
a division of Penguin Books USA Inc.

10 9 8 7 6 5 4 3 2 1

PUBLISHER'S NOTE
The ideas, procedures, and suggestions contained in this book are not
intended as a substitute for consulting with your physician. All matters
regarding your health require medical supervision.

Grateful acknowledgment is made for permission to reprint "Seasoning
with Herbs and Spices" by Fran Rukenbrod. By permission of the author.

LIBRARY OF CONGRESS CATALOGING-IN-PUBLICATION DATA

Schwab, Steven.
    Eating well, living well with kidney disease / by Steven Schwab and
  Dorothy Bartholomay ; with Michelle McGee.
      p.   cm.
    Includes bibliographical references and index.
    ISBN 0-670-86633-4 (alk. paper)
    1. Kidneys—Diseases—Nutritional aspects.   2. Kidneys—Diseases—
  Diet therapy.   I. Bartholomay, Dorothy.   II. McGee, Michelle.
  III. Title.
  RC903.S38   1997
  616.6′10654—dc20   96–27911

This book is printed on acid-free paper.

∞

Printed in the United States of America
Set in Minion

Contents

Foreword

Good nutrition is the cornerstone of good health. At the Sarah W. Stedman Center for Nutritional Studies, we are committed to the idea that optimum health care includes comprehensive nutritional care. At the Nutrition Center, we routinely incorporate the results of research studies on nutrition and disease into the medical/health-care plans of our patients.

The purpose of the *Eating Well, Living Well* series is to share the expert knowledge of the medical doctors and nutritionists who work within the Duke Medical Center community at the level of nutritional therapy and lifestyle intervention. Education is the key to the prevention and treatment of many common diseases. Yet much of the information available today about nutrition and diet is incomplete and/or inaccurate. We hope that the *Eating Well, Living Well* series will begin to resolve some of the controversies associated with present-day diets.

Many popularly promoted diets are not founded on sound nutritional principles and common sense. Such diets are difficult for most people to follow, usually because there is no consideration for those with special health concerns. That is why we include in each book sections on selecting the right foods in a variety of settings, including grocery stores, restaurants, and recreational events. Another problem with catch-all and fad diets is that there are often no special considerations for individual differences in activity, age, or lifestyle.

The *Eating Well, Living Well* series addresses these issues directly. We have asked experts from specific fields of clinical research and practice to write about disease prevention by nutritional means, with specific emphasis on individual differences and exceptions to the rules. Each book is uniquely tailored for each disease. This book explores the latest nutritional aspects of kidney disease, a progressive condition that affects the delicate balance of fluids, minerals, and waste products in the body.

Sarah White Stedman

Acknowledgments

Thanks to our families for understanding our passion for our work on kidney disease. Special thanks to Patty Yunker, Research Chef at the Sarah W. Stedman Center for Nutritional Studies, for her guidance and creativity in preparing the recipes for this book.

Chapter One

What Is Kidney Disease?

I f you picked up this book, you are probably one of the thousands of people who have kidney disease and have been told by their physician to follow a better diet or a special diet. Now you are asking why and especially how; how, really, do you expect me to do it? We want to put the special diet you have been prescribed within your reach. And we want to show you that, in fact, you can do it, and it will improve the way you feel.

This book is about giving you the facts that the medical community has come to know about kidney disease, nutrition, and health. It is also important to say what this book is not. It is not a description of a fad diet or a diet based on a commercial product. It is not a weight-loss diet, though it can be adapted, when appropriate, for people with kidney disease who also need to lose weight. It is a diet only because it describes an entire system for choosing foods, for deciding what is best to eat.

Please note that this book does not include specific recommendations for children or vegetarians with kidney disease or for people who have already had a successful kidney transplant. Children have the added challenge of constant growth; vegetarians' protein requirements must be approached differently; and kidney transplant recipients have widely varying levels of kidney function, making it difficult to generalize about their dietary needs. To find out how you can adapt this book's program to special needs such as these, consult your physician or a dietitian who specializes in kidney disease.

In recent years, medical research has begun to focus on the relationship between what people eat and what diseases they get, and how these diseases progress. The diet in this book is based on medical knowledge, and that knowledge is based on the currently well-established dietary treatment of kidney disease.

How can you make this knowledge work for you? Use the book as an evaluation tool, to take stock of what you know; to find out what questions you need to ask. This book is not meant as a substitute for medical advice you receive from your family doctor, kidney specialist, or dietitian; the facts we present here are an adjunct to that advice. It is our hope that you will involve your health-care providers in your efforts to change your diet and lifestyle.

Try the kidney-smart recipes, and experiment with other recipes you find. The recipes are meant to help you on your way to following the diet recommendations. Registered dietitians in particular are trained to answer practical questions about diet and can serve a very useful role in your reaching your goal to change your diet. A number of other important resources—organizations and publications—are listed at the end of the book.

The Kidneys

Most people have two kidneys, each varying in size from 3 to 7 inches in length; to imagine their shape, think of a kidney bean. They are located near the spine midway down the back, one on the right and one on the left.

The word **renal** is often used when describing something that relates to the kidneys, as in the phrase "renal nutrition." "Ren-" is the Greek prefix for kidney. In Latin, the prefix is "nephr-," as in **nephrologist**, or kidney doctor.

Today, approximately 10 percent of the American population is born with or has only one functioning kidney. In these cases, the functioning kidney usually becomes larger than average to compensate for the damaged or missing one. Adequate kidney function is a priority, and the body puts much effort into maintaining it.

Why are the kidneys so important? The kidneys regulate salt and water balance and eliminate toxins from the blood. They have the unique ability to maintain the concentrations of the chemicals in our blood within fairly narrow limits, allowing our body to function at maximum efficiency. The kidneys perform these functions by filtering the blood—all 5 or so liters of it every 45 to 60 minutes—and selectively reclaiming those substances that are needed, excreting those that are not. Each kidney houses millions of intricate filters, called **nephrons**. The nephrons serve to separate out the blood's fluid portion, then to further separate the fluid into a part to keep and a part to get rid of. The kidneys get rid of the unwanted substances—toxins, extra minerals, and extra water— through urine. In this way, the kidneys are like traffic police, directing the flow of these substances out of the body.

When Kidneys Fail

Kidney disease is a condition in which the kidneys slowly or suddenly lose the ability to do their job. A sudden loss of kidney function, termed **acute renal failure**, can occur when the kidneys are subjected to a sudden shock that forces them to "turn off" in order to survive. A common cause of acute renal failure is very low blood pressure, such as occurs when someone loses a significant amount of blood, perhaps in an accident. In these cases, the kidneys almost always recover in two to three weeks, when overall health returns. Acute renal failure rarely leads to long-term kidney failure.

In contrast, diseases such as **diabetes mellitus** (see below, under Causes of Kidney Failure) can permanently damage the kidneys. Permanent damage results in **chronic renal failure**—chronic because it continues over a long period of time. **Renal insufficiency**, when the kidneys are not functioning at a normal level but are still capable of sustaining most bodily functions, is characteristic of this condition. By following the special diet outlined in this book and taking appropriate medications, health can be maintained in those with renal insufficiency even though their kidneys are diseased.

When kidney disease progresses to less than 5 percent of normal kidney function, a period of dependence on an artificial kidney is begun. Use of an artificial kidney is called **renal replacement therapy**. It is also known by the common term **dialysis**. Without medical intervention a person with so-called **end-stage renal disease** or **dialysis-dependent renal failure** would not be able to survive long.

Dialysis can be accomplished two different ways. The most common type is **hemodialysis**. "Heme" means blood in Latin; hemodialysis directly involves the blood. Blood from veins in the arms or chest is transferred outside the body, through an artificial kidney composed of layers of selectively permeable plastic membranes, then, within moments, the "cleaned" blood is returned to the body. Cleaning all the blood in the body takes about three to four hours, and it is usually recommended that the entire treatment be done three times per week. Hemodialysis is always supervised and, therefore, is typically done in special facilities. Willing partners can be trained to perform hemodialysis in the home.

The other type of renal replacement therapy, called **peritoneal dialysis**, is becoming more common. **Peritoneum** is another word for the inside wall of the abdomen. In this method, fluid containing dextrose, a kind of sugar, is placed inside the abdomen—in the cavity surrounding the organs—via a tube through the abdominal wall. The peritoneum acts as a filter, allowing toxins, extra minerals, and fluid to pass into the dextrose solution, where they are held until the solution is drained off. Peritoneal dialysis can be performed with daily exchanges at home or elsewhere, which allows for flexibility in a person's routine. These exchanges can also be done at night during sleeping hours with the aid of a machine.

The role of dialysis is to maintain a basal level of kidney function through artificial means. *All types of treatment for kidney failure require modifications of diet and medications to accommodate artificial rather than natural kidney function.*

Causes of Kidney Failure

In the United States the most common cause of kidney failure is diabetes mellitus, both insulin-dependent and noninsulin-dependent. The second most common cause of kidney failure is damage from long-standing high blood pressure, also called **hypertension**. Other common causes include a class of diseases called glomerulonephritides. These diseases involve damage to the filters of the kidneys. Other causes are inherited, such as polycystic kidney diseases, or acquired, such as by overexposure to toxins from certain drugs. Regardless of the cause of kidney failure, medical treatment is much the same.

Measuring Kidney Function

Physicians can measure kidney function in many different ways. The actual size of the kidney is important but does not provide much information on the level of kidney function, which can only be measured by looking at toxins in the blood and at the urinary excretion of certain substances. Physicians determine your kidney function by analyzing samples of your blood and urine, which are often taken over a period of time.

In the blood, levels of **creatinine** and **blood urea nitrogen** (BUN) are the two most important indicators of renal function. (Urea is an unusable protein byproduct.) Creatinine is a compound that is released by all the body's muscles at a steady rate. Once released, it is rapidly excreted by the kidneys. Build-up of serum creatinine above normal levels signals impaired kidney function, and, naturally, the greater the build-up the worse the kidneys' condition. Usually, when serum creatinine reaches 7 in diabetics and 10 in nondiabetics some form of dialysis therapy is required.

BUN reflects the breakdown of proteins by the body. High BUN usually results from the kidneys not being able to get rid of waste protein in the blood. Doctors, nurses, and dietitians monitor this blood level and use it as a guideline in adjusting your diet recommendations, medications, and course of dialysis.

An even more exact measure of kidney function is creatinine excretion in the urine over 24 hours. This measurement is termed **creatinine clearance** and is more accurate than levels of serum creatinine or BUN.

There are also special nuclear medicine tests that accurately measure kidney function by determining kidney blood flow and the kidney's ability to excrete radioactive substances injected into the bloodstream. While accurate, these tests are very expensive and are only used occasionally. Studies involving contrast or dye injected into the bloodstream are rarely done in renal failure because of the possibility that the dye may further damage the kidneys.

Occasionally a procedure termed **ultrasound** is necessary to make sure that symptoms of renal failure are not being caused or worsened by a blockage to urine flow (such as a kidney stone). Ultrasound is harmless; it uses sound waves to make a picture of your kidneys.

Preventing Loss of Kidney Function

Some types of kidney disease can be prevented altogether, and most types can be slowed down. Recent evidence shows that tight control of blood sugar in insulin-dependent (Type I) diabetes can slow or prevent the progression of kidney disease. In addition, most kidney disease is slowed down dramatically when blood pressure is restored to normal levels (120 / 80 mmHg is normal). *Regardless of the underlying disease, changes in diet and exercise and the use of medications to treat high blood pressure and diabetes will slow the progression of kidney disease.* Working with your physician and dietitian to control these factors has been shown to be very beneficial. Don't ignore this good news.

Altered Drug Metabolism in Kidney Disease

It is important for anyone with kidney disease to pay careful attention to medication. Many prescription and over-the-counter medications are excreted by the kidneys; when your kidneys are not functioning fully they may have trouble getting rid of them. When medications build up in the body they can become toxic. Any medication that is normally excreted by the kidneys must be taken in reduced amounts, discontinued, or avoided by people with kidney disease. Ask your physician. Even the metabolism of the diabetes medicine insulin is affected by kidney disease, so you should talk to your physician about reevaluating your insulin needs. **Remember: Dosages for any medications you take must be determined by a physician.**

Vitamin and Mineral Supplements

Vitamin and mineral supplements have become popular "health products." Though the jury is still out on just how beneficial many of the supplements are in preventing disease, many people (including some health professionals) continue to use supplements. And for most people that's okay, because there is little chance that most supplements will do any harm.

This is *not* so for people with diseased kidneys. In much the same way that the metabolism of certain medications is altered with renal disease, vitamin and mineral metabolism is also disrupted. **You should take supplements only by prescription or with your physician's approval.** Even a general multivitamin is a mixed bag of substances, some potentially beneficial and others potentially toxic, when kidney function is compromised.

On the other hand, medically approved vitamin and mineral supplements can be of great benefit to your health. Calcium supplementation, for example, is a necessity for most people with renal failure. In fact, supplemental calcium is sometimes given straight into the bloodstream. Without it, bone disease would develop.

Other supplements that are commonly prescribed for people with kidney disease include the mineral iron and some of the B vitamins. Again, the bottom line is that you need to talk to your physician or dietitian about vitamin and mineral supplements before you take them.

Chapter Two

Good Nutrition for Your Kidneys

What you eat affects how you and your kidneys work: This is a medical fact. It may not seem like a huge discovery, but the way better nutrition works to improve health is increasingly being viewed as a wonder of medicine.

Eating a diet that contains controlled amounts of protein and restricted amounts of sodium, potassium, and phosphorus (see next three chapters) lessens the workload of the kidneys. When stress and strain are removed from the kidneys, their condition improves. Most important, though, by restricting your diet you allow fewer substances that are toxic to your kidneys to be introduced into your body. Fewer waste products build up, and you avoid or alleviate the often unpleasant and even dangerous symptoms and outcomes of kidney disease. Your kidneys won't have to work so hard trying to take the toxins out if you don't let them in! This is the medical wonder. It is that simple.

Controlling and restricting food intake is not all that simple. But don't be afraid to change. We want to help you make the dietary changes that will allow you to prolong the natural life of your kidneys. For those who are already receiving dialysis therapy and for those who would like to forgo dialysis for as long as possible, there is considerable evidence that following a diet like the one described in this book—one tailor-made for your condition—will improve your health.

Food Guide Pyramid

Today, the compositional starting point for all diets is the Food Guide Pyramid. First, the majority of what a person eats should be starchy foods—breads, cereals, pastas, and rice. Second, one's diet should contain generous amounts of fruits and vegetables. Third, meats and other high-protein foods should be included in one's diet but only in carefully chosen, somewhat limited amounts. Last, added fats and simple sugars should be used sparingly so as to make up only a very small part of one's overall diet.

The Food Guide Pyramids below represent an average best diet. (Think of meeting the criteria *on average, over time.* No one balances his or her diet perfectly all of the time.) The Stedman Center recommends to people receiving dialysis treatments a diet that corresponds to that depicted in the first Food Guide Pyramid (page 12). This pyramid corresponds to the nationally recognized Food Guide Pyramid for healthy persons.

Presented in the second of the two Food Guide Pyramids (page 13) is a variation that depicts the protein-restricted diet recommended for people with renal insufficiency who are not yet being treated with dialysis.

In the protein-restriction version, the protein and dairy sections have been cut in half. To compensate and make the diet whole again, all of the remaining sections have been enlarged. Thus **the protein-restricted diet contains increased amounts of carbohydrates, fruits, vegetables, and, to a lesser extent, added fats and significantly**

The Food Guide Pyramid: Diet Recommendations for People with Kidney Disease

For Those on Dialysis Treatments

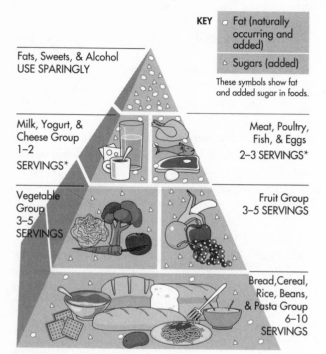

KEY
- Fat (naturally occurring and added)
- Sugars (added)

These symbols show fat and added sugar in foods.

Fats, Sweets, & Alcohol
USE SPARINGLY

Milk, Yogurt, & Cheese Group
1–2 SERVINGS*

Meat, Poultry, Fish, & Eggs
2–3 SERVINGS*

Vegetable Group
3–5 SERVINGS

Fruit Group
3–5 SERVINGS

Bread, Cereal, Rice, Beans, & Pasta Group
6–10 SERVINGS

*See the table on p. 64 for recommended servings according to your protein requirement, given on p. 28 or p. 32.

less protein-rich meats and dairy products when compared to the dialysis diet.

In both cases, the carbohydrate section and the fat section, at the very top and the very bottom, can be shifted in size. The pyramid is flexible in that way. The sizes of the protein section and the dairy section, on the other hand, have to be rigidly set because protein malnu-

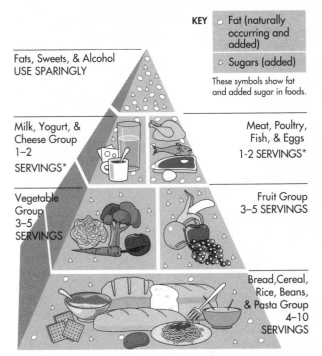

KEY
- Fat (naturally occurring and added)
- Sugars (added)

These symbols show fat and added sugar in foods.

Fats, Sweets, & Alcohol
USE SPARINGLY

Milk, Yogurt, & Cheese Group
1–2 SERVINGS*

Meat, Poultry, Fish, & Eggs
1-2 SERVINGS*

Vegetable Group
3–5 SERVINGS

Fruit Group
3–5 SERVINGS

Bread, Cereal, Rice, Beans, & Pasta Group
4–10 SERVINGS

*See the table on p. 64 for recommended servings according to your protein requirement, given on p. 28 or p. 32.

trition is the direct cause of many of the health problems associated with renal disease.

In Chapter Six, Meal Planning, we will show you how to apply the ideals contained in the Food Guide Pyramid to what you eat.

A Word About Diabetes

Diabetes is a disease that many of you with kidney disease have been living with for a long time. With diabetes there is an entire set of nutritional guidelines that are prescribed, usually from very early on. The guidelines, which include restriction of sugar and fat, were designed to moderate blood sugar levels and prevent early development of heart disease and renal disease.

Once your kidneys fail, the treatment of your diabetes will change, including changing your diet to meet renal diet restrictions. You will not need to "forget" all that you learned about diabetes nutrition. What you have already learned will just help you understand the renal diet guidelines better. Because you have or are close to kidney failure, following the renal diet with special consideration for saturated fat and sugar intake is what will best address your immediate health concerns. Renal failure is a serious development for a person with diabetes. With it, it becomes even more critical that you monitor and restrict your diet.

The Value of Food

The purpose of eating is to nourish the body. How is the value of food to the body measured? One measure is how much energy is released when the food is burned, or metabolized. This measure, called **calories,** tells us about the **energetic value** of food. Protein, fat, carbohydrate, and alcohol all have energetic value. All foods are made up of at least one of the first three of these components, and most are a combination. These energy substances are called **macronutrients**. How many calories there are per gram of each is shown below.

Carbohydrate = 4 calories/gram*
Protein = 4 calories/gram
Fat = 9 calories/gram
Alcohol = 7 calories/gram

A copper penny weighs about one gram.

Carbohydrate comes in two forms: simple and complex. Simple carbohydrates are what you think of as sugar; complex carbohydrates are often called starches. In addition to plain sugar, simple carbohydrates are found naturally in fruits and fruit juices and are added to most regular sodas and sweets. Complex carbohydrates are found in pastas, breads, cereals, and vegetables. Many foods that are naturally high in carbohydrates, such as whole grain foods, fruits, vegetables, and beans, also contain **fiber,** an important food substance that aids in digestion.

Major sources of **protein** in the diet are red meats, poultry, seafood, eggs, dairy products, organ meats, nuts, and dry beans (though the latter three should be avoided by people with kidney disease). Protein is required for building strong muscles, skin, bone, and hair. Like a beaded necklace or a length of chain, protein is made of subunits, called amino acids, that are strung together. Several specific amino acids cannot be made by our own bodies and must therefore be taken in through the food we eat. These amino acids are called **essential**—it is essential that you eat them. This is not difficult if you follow a properly balanced diet like the one outlined here.

Fat is what you see when you look at a pat of butter or margarine or a spoonful of oil. What makes some fat solid and other fat liquid is the degree of **saturation**. In general, solid fats must be used more sparingly than liquid fats, because they are more saturated. Margarine is the exception. It is solid but contains mostly unsaturated fats. Saturated fats are linked to raising blood cholesterol levels. Meats and dairy products contain varying amounts of fat, mostly saturated. Today, lean meats and low-fat dairy products are increasingly recommended for reducing saturated fat intake. Sandwich spreads, salad dressings, and nuts also contain a fair amount of fat, but it is mostly unsaturated. Fat occupies the topmost and, therefore, narrowest part of the Food Guide Pyramid. Fats are a rich source of calories and, under normal circumstances, have to be moderated to keep you from exceeding your energy needs.

Alcohol also provides your body with some energy, but it should not make up a significant portion of anyone's daily calories. Its calories have no other nutritional value, and its metabolism can interfere with the treatment of your disease. You should consult your physician about inclusion of alcohol in your diet. If it is allowed, a dietitian can help you fit it into your meal plans.

There are also important **micronutrients**—vitamins and minerals—as well as fiber that are present in foods and contribute to their **overall nutritional value**. Therefore, we must be aware of the added value of certain foods. Whole foods, or foods that have not been processed prior to your using them, generally have higher added value than processed foods. This is because processing methods tend to destroy or remove the micronutrients and fiber naturally present in many foods. In general, the more whole, unprocessed foods you eat, the more good micronutrients you will get.

Food Metabolism: You Are What You Eat

Many of the calories and, thus, macronutrients that we eat each day are used up quickly by the billions of hungry cells in our body. That's why we usually eat several meals a day. And like a retail store that keeps back stock on certain items, our body stores the major macronutrients so that even when we have not recently eaten we can have some energy.

Carbohydrate is dedicated exclusively to providing energy needed to walk, talk, think, hum, swim, and generally get around. The liver maintains a generous reserve of carbohydrate when it can. If you do not get enough calories from carbohydrate each day, your body will use up the liver's store quickly. Extra carbohydrate is occasionally made into and stored as fat. Virtually no carbohydrate is normally gotten rid of by the body—it is all used. That is how much the body depends on this macronutrient.

The body is more discriminating when it comes to protein, though not less dependent on it. A small amount of protein normally circulates in the blood. From there it is stored in muscle and available to other cells that need it to function. As the level of protein in the blood increases, it is the kidneys' job to get rid of the extra, which is first converted into the unusable protein byproduct urea. Of course, when the kidneys fail, urea cannot be excreted and so builds up in the blood. The condition of too much protein waste in the blood is called **uremia**. Symptoms of uremia include loss of appetite, nausea and vomiting, muscle cramps, foul breath, trouble concentrating, and, occasionally, tremors.

So where does fat fit into this complex metabolic picture? Fat, another major macronutrient, makes the body run smoothly—literally like a well-oiled engine. A fair amount of fat has to be included in your diet to maintain proper functioning. In addition to helping things run smoothly, fat can, at times, be broken down and used as energy. And a power-packed energy it is. Under the right circumstances, with over twice the energy per gram as protein or carbohydrate, fat provides concentrated energy. Fat-provided energy, however, does not make you feel superhuman. The point is that a little bit of fat goes a long way. Overall, dietary fat, when part of a healthy diet and lifestyle, is beneficial to health. The other side of the dietary fat coin is heart disease and obesity.

Heart disease is like engine failure. It develops when the heart, which is the engine's motor, is filled with mucky oil and then put under stress for a long period of time. Many factors influence the development of heart disease, including the make of the car (genetics), the type of stress it is under (driving in the Indy 500 versus driving to work), and the type of oil in the motor—which brings us back to nutrition. There are three broad categories of "oil," or fat, in your diet. They are saturated, monounsaturated, and polyunsaturated. Again, saturated fats are the least desirable and are the ones most often associated with development of heart disease. For people with high cholesterol, saturated fat intake should be minimized. Easy ways to avoid extra saturated fat are to trim the visible fat from meats, choose margarine or vegetable oil over butter, and reduce the amount of high-fat cheese you eat.

Many people suffer from both heart disease and renal failure, and need nutritional advice tailored to their unique circumstances. We strongly recommend discussing concerns about your diet with your physician and perhaps seeking a nutritional consultation with a dietitian. We recommend a similar course of action for people who have renal disease and are obese.

Calorie Requirement and Weight Loss

Energy input equals energy output is the mantra for understanding daily calorie requirements. Energy input is determined, essentially, by the food you eat. Energy output, on the other hand, is affected by many factors, the most important being your exercise pattern and rate of metabolism.

If you are exercising or working vigorously you expend a great deal of energy, so you must replace it with an equal amount of food energy to balance the equation. If you are inactive, then you burn a basal (but nonetheless substantial) amount of energy during your normal activities. For the most part, the less active you are the lower your calorie requirement, but factors such as genetics, the added physical and mental stress of having a disease, and disease treatment in the case of dialysis may increase your basal level so that you have to eat more than you think you do in order to maintain your weight.

Daily Calorie Requirement According to Body Weight Goal	
Body weight (lbs.)	Range for Daily Calorie Intake (Min. for Peritoneal Dialysis)
110	(1,250) 1,500–1,750
120	(1,350) 1,650–1,900
130	(1,500) 1,800–2,050
140	(1,600) 1,900–2,250
150	(1,700) 2,050–2,400
160	(1,800) 2,200–2,550
170	(1,950) 2,300–2,700
180	(2,050) 2,450–2,850
190	(2,150) 2,600–3,000
200	(2,250) 2,750–3,200

The calories given in parentheses are the lower limit for a person on peritoneal dialysis.

A chart of healthy body weight goals can be found on page 85.

If you are very active, the number of calories you will need to maintain or reach a healthy body weight will be toward the higher end of the range given for that weight. If you are not active, aim for the value at the lower end of the range. The number of calories people on peritoneal dialysis need is slightly lower than others', and so a lower minimum (in parentheses) is specified for them. (The dextrose solution used during peritoneal dialysis treatments contains calories in the form of simple sugars.) Keep in mind that the calorie recommendations we have provided here do not override any given to you by your physician or dietitian.

Overweight is associated with increased morbidity in those with kidney and other types of diseases. Thus weight loss can be a valuable goal for many people with kidney disease, and the earlier in your disease you reach a healthy body weight, the better. Losing weight means changing the mantra from the same amount of energy input and output to **more energy output than input.** This means exercising or being generally more active, plus eating less. To determine a daily calorie goal for losing weight, first find your healthy weight (page 85). Then, find the number of calories required for your *healthy* weight in the table above.

If you are more than 20 percent over your healthy weight, we recommend reducing your calorie intake *incrementally.* Don't try to do it all at once! For instance, aim for and reach the goal of being within 10 percent of your healthy weight before losing more. Gradual weight loss of not more than two pounds a week is more healthy than rapid weight loss, and the losses are more likely to be sustainable. In general, we also recommend that people who are more than 20 percent over their healthy weight get nutritional counseling about weight loss. The malnutrition that can occur with unhealthy weight reduction can, in some cases, further damage the kidneys or other organs.

Once end-stage renal disease is reached, a more pressing goal than reaching an ideal body weight is getting *enough* calories and other nutrients to maintain good health. People who are on dialysis and not obese should, for the most part, look at their calorie requirement not as a limitation but as an invitation to eat enough food to meet their body's needs. At the end of the next chapter we discuss easy ways to increase your calorie intake if this applies to you.

Nutrition Labels

In the last several years great strides have been made in getting food companies to pay attention to nutrition. Federal regulations requiring that all manufactured foods and beverages have nutrition labels are now in place. Giving consumers the option to make informed food choices by reading labels is a step in the right direction.

Nutrition labels are your eyes into the composition of food. They tell you what the box, bag, jar, jug, package, or can you are looking at contains. Sure it's cottage cheese, but what's in cottage cheese?

Key information provided on nutrition labels:

- *Serving size* and *number of servings*. Tells you what amount of the item in the package the information on the label applies to. The information on the label only occasionally refers to what is in the whole package; and often the serving size that the information on the label describes is *considerably less* than what the typical person would eat at one time. In the example of cottage cheese, eating ½ of a cup

Sample Nutrition Label
Cottage Cheese, 1% Low-fat

Nutrition Facts

Serving Size ¼ cup (48 g)
Servings Per Container 4

Amount Per Serving

Calories 41   Calories from Fat 9

% Daily Value*

Total Fat 1 g	**2%**
Saturated Fat 0.5 g	**2%**
Cholesterol 2.5 mg	**1%**
Sodium 230 mg	**10%**
Total Carbohydrate 1.5 g	**1%**
Dietary Fiber 0 g	**0%**
Sugars 0 g	
Protein 7 g	

Vitamin A	1%	•	Vitamin C	0%
Calcium	4%	•	Iron	4%

* Percent Daily Values are based on a 2,000
calorie diet. Your daily values may be higher or
lower depending on your calorie needs:

	Calories	2,000	2,600
Total Fat	Less than	65 g	80 g
Sat. Fat	Less than	20 g	25 g
Cholesterol	Less than	300 mg	300 mg
Sodium	Less than	2,400 mg	2,400 mg
Total Carbohydrate		300 g	375 g
Fiber		25 g	30 g

Calories per gram:
Fat 9   •   Carbohydrate 4   •   Protein 4

More nutrients may be listed on some labels.

of cottage cheese is not unreasonable, yet you must be aware that the information on the label describes only a ¼-cup serving. Therefore, you would get twice as much of everything if you ate a ½-cup serving. That would be 82 calories, 2 g of fat, 14 g of protein, 460 g of sodium, etc.

- *Calories.* Tells you the energetic value of the food. Remember, this is calories per serving.
- *Fat (and saturated fat), protein, carbohydrate (and sugar).* Tells you the amount of each macronutrient, measured in grams (g). Knowing the protein content will help you properly monitor the protein in your diet. In looking at fat content, choose foods with the least amount of fat as saturated fat.
- *Sodium.* Measured in milligrams (mg). In general, minimize the amount you eat by limiting the amount in any one food to 250 mg per serving. Again, if you are going to eat more than one serving, you must factor that in.
- *Vitamins and minerals.* In general, the more the better. You have to be careful with vitamins and mineral supplements, but the vitamins and minerals provided in ordinary foods are okay.

Chapter Three

Protein

For anyone with kidney disease, protein is the cornerstone of your diet. For some that means properly restricting it; others must make sure they get enough. Managing dietary protein encompasses two ideals. One is getting the right amount. The other is getting the right kind.

Protein Quality

Sources of protein can be divided into two broad categories: high-quality and low-quality. Quality, in the case of protein, refers to the number of different types of amino acids the food contains. High-quality protein foods contain a wide variety of amino acids, and they are present in the optimum proportions. Because of their richness, high-quality protein sources are more desirable for a renal diet. Low-quality protein foods contain only a limited number of types of amino acid and are, therefore, incomplete. The protein from low-quality sources is more likely to be converted into urea and not utilized for building muscle tissue.

We recommend that at least 60 to 70 percent of the protein you eat be of high quality. To imagine this relationship, think of spending money. Say you take $100 out of the bank. We are asking that you spend no more than $40 of it on knickknacks and other "nonessentials" and at least $60 of it doing and buying only the essential things.

Focus on these good sources of high-quality protein.	Eat these foods moderately. They contain some low-quality protein.	Avoid these foods! They contain lots of low-quality protein.
Beef	Bran cereals	*Nuts & butters*
Pork	Whole wheat breads	Peanut
Chicken	Bran muffins	Cashew
Turkey	Granola	Walnut
Fish	Lima beans	Pistachio
Eggs	Broccoli	Pecan
Shrimp	Spinach	Almond
Oysters	Greens	Chestnut
Dairy products	Brussels sprouts	
Wild game	Potatoes (always eat	*Dried beans/peas*
Soybeans/tofu*	without the skin)	Black-eyed peas
		Kidney/pinto beans
		Lentils
		Split peas

*This is an exception to the rule that dried beans and peas should be avoided.

Good sources of high-quality protein should be an integral part of your diet. Even for people following a protein-restricted diet, these same choices are appropriate, just in lesser amounts.

All dairy products contain high-quality protein. To a small extent, ice cream, yogurt, sour cream, cream cheese, and milk can be included in your diet. On the other hand, cheeses (other than cottage and cream) as well as processed meats, such as deli, canned, or smoked meats, that are not specially made to be low in sodium should not be eaten. Though they contain high-quality protein, they are high in sodium (see Chapter Four), a mineral that will strain your already aching kidneys. Organ meats contain high-quality protein but should not be included in your diet because they contain substances that are undesirable for renal diets.

Low-quality protein is present in the highest concentrations in dried beans and dried peas. We recommend you cut these sources of low-quality protein from your diet altogether. Nuts and nut butters need to be greatly limited in your diet for the same reason.

Whole grain cereals and breads and certain vegetables contain some protein, and it is low quality. But both whole grain products and vegetables also contain fiber and vitamins and minerals that increase their overall nutritional value. Whole grain products and high-protein vegetables such as those listed in the table on page 25 should not make up a staple in your diet, but they can be eaten occasionally or whenever you can fit them nutritionally into your meal plans (see Chapter Six).

Protein Restriction: Preventing Kidney Failure, Living Without Dialysis

Note: Skip to the next section (beginning on page 31) if you are on dialysis.

By getting sick your kidneys are telling you they need a break from the stress and strain of filtering, which is what they do all day and all night. When you are in the beginning stages of kidney disease and not on dialysis, it is imperative that you limit the amount of protein in your diet, because all the extra protein you eat has to be eliminated by the kidneys. Restrict the protein you eat and you help your kidneys by acting like a filter for them—getting rid of the protein before it even gets into your body. *Your diet works in place of your kidneys,* relieving some of the strain on them. Make appropriate low-protein food choices, and you can prolong the health of your kidneys and may even delay the need for dialysis.

Certainly, though, eliminating every last bit of protein from your diet would also have potentially unhealthy consequences. Examples of drastic protein-restriction diets do exist and have been shown to afford moderate benefits for certain patients with kidney disease. But on the whole, individuals following such diets are at increased risk for various nutritional deficiencies, the syndromes they cause, and muscle wasting. Thus the diet recommended by the Stedman Center and outlined here contains a moderate but restricted amount of protein and is in accord with the guidelines offered by the American Dietetic Association and other organizations concerned with renal nutrition and health. This diet has been shown to minimize uremic symptoms and maintain proper nutritional balance when followed closely.

To determine your daily protein requirement, find your body weight goal in the far left column of the table on page 28. As you go across the table to the right, the first column you come to gives you a range for how many grams of protein you should eat each day. (Nutrition labels and most cookbooks that offer nutritional information list protein content in grams, the unit we have used here.)

The next column in the table gives a range for the minimum number of grams of protein (60 percent of the total) that should be of high quality. To get the number of grams of low-quality protein allowed, subtract this number from the number in the previous column. The quality

Predialysis Diet: Daily Protein Restriction According to Body Weight Goal*

Body weight (lbs.)	Total Daily Protein Intake Range	Minimum (60 Percent of Total) High-Quality Protein Intake Range
120	32–43	19–26
130	35–47	21–28
140	38–50	23–30
150	41–54	24–32
160	43–58	26–35
170	46–61	28–37
180	49–65	29–39
190	51–68	31–41
200	54–72	32–43

*Healthy body weights are listed on page 85.

of the protein in a food is rarely indicated on a label or in a nutritional analysis. It is your task to make that assessment.

So what do these numbers mean in terms of food? We'll begin with the fact that there are about 7 grams of high-quality protein in 1 ounce of cooked meat, poultry, or seafood, ¼ cup of cottage cheese, or one egg. Therefore, to meet a daily high-quality protein requirement of, for example, 28 grams, you would need to eat *no more than* 4 ounces of cooked meat (4 × 7 g = 28 g), or the equivalent, each day. A typical serving of cooked meat is 3 ounces, about the size of a deck of cards (more at restaurants). You could meet that requirement by having one larger-than-average serving of meat at one meal or by having two very small servings at two meals. You can vary your strategy from day to day.

In addition to meat, you get high-quality protein—about 4 grams per serving—from dairy products. A serving equals ½ cup of milk, sour cream, or yogurt or ⅔ cup of ice cream. Dairy products are restricted in the renal diet, though, because they contain significant amounts of the several minerals that can cause trouble for people with kidney disease. In general, limit yourself to 1 dairy serving each day.

To ensure that you always know how much protein you are getting, we recommend that you weigh out the meat portions you eat. Small kitchen balances can be purchased at stores carrying kitchenware. The serving size amounts and grams given here for meat are based on the cooked weight. If you are preparing a mixed dish, you can weigh according to the weight of the raw meat, but you should increase the weight by one-quarter. For instance, if you want 3 ounces cooked you should start with 4 ounces raw. Refer to page 70 for a formula for converting cooked and raw meat weights.

If you try to restrict your protein by eliminating high-quality protein such as meats and eggs altogether, you run the risk of protein malnutrition. You will likely not get sufficient amounts of the amino acids that are essential to your health.

In general, it is difficult for a person who has to eat less than about 50 grams of protein per day to get enough high-quality protein without exceeding their daily total protein limit. If you are concerned about or know you are not getting all the high-quality protein you need or are constantly exceeding your protein restriction, you can integrate special low-protein versions of normal food ingredients, including flours, pastas, and dairy products, into your diet. Low-protein products are available from specialty stores and through mail-order catalogs. Nondairy creamers are available at many grocery stores in the dairy case. In the Resources section in the back of this book we provide information on companies that make low-protein and other diet specialty products. Many companies will also make available recipes that utilize their products.

Those of you on protein-restricted diets must constantly balance your "protein bank account." The better your kidneys function, the more money you have in the bank. The more your kidneys are failing, the more you must be aware of how you "spend" every gram of protein, just as you are more aware of how you spend money when you have a limited amount in the bank. Easing your kidney disease is a matter of saving. And as with money, after a time you become more "frugal"; with protein, that means that eating less becomes more natural.

A good place to begin learning protein frugality is the first meal of the day, breakfast. Instead of having a scrambled egg, sausage patties, and toast (protein = 20 g), have grits or oatmeal and a slice of toast or an English muffin with your favorite jam (protein = 6 g). Or have a slice of French toast topped with warm fruit compote (protein = 6 g). It's an easy meal to pull together and is very tasty and satisfying. Pancakes are another satisfying low-protein breakfast option, but watch out for sodium and phosphorus in store-bought mixes and syrups.

In addition to meatless breakfasts, many people on protein restriction need to have one other meatless meal each day. Again, once you get in the habit and learn to enjoy more breads, cereals, fruits, and vegetables, protein restriction will get easier.

We encourage you to keep a running balance of the protein in your account. As with your bank account, if you do not keep a running record of what you eat *and* record the protein values on a continual basis so that you can see how much you have left, you will constantly over-draw on your protein account. (See the table on page 61 for the average protein values of foods, and the ones on pages 66–69 for low-protein sample food records.)

Protein Requirements When on Dialysis

Note: Skip this section if you are not on dialysis.

The need for protein goes back up from the protein restriction of renal insufficiency to a normal level once you begin dialysis therapy. Dialysis treatments are very effective at filtering protein waste from the blood, and in fact they usually go a little overboard, removing some viable amino acids with each treatment. Getting an adequate amount of protein is the goal.

To determine your daily protein requirement, find your body weight goal in the far left column of the table on page 32. Going across the table to the right, the first column you come to gives you a range for how many grams of protein you should eat each day. (Grams, the unit we have used here, is the way that protein is listed on nutrition labels and the way most cookbooks that offer nutritional information list protein content.)

The next column you come to shows the minimum number of grams of protein (60 percent of the total) that should be of high quality. To get the number of grams of low-quality protein allowed, subtract this number from the number in the previous column. The quality of the protein in a food is rarely indicated on a label or in a nutritional analysis. It is your task to make that assessment.

So what do these numbers mean in terms of food?

Dialysis Diet: Daily Protein Requirement According to Body Weight Goal.*

Body weight (lbs.)	Total Daily Protein Range for Intake (Max. for Peritoneal Dialysis)	Minimum (60 Percent of Total) High-Quality Protein Intake Range
120	55–66 (72)	33–40 (43)
130	59–71 (77)	35–43 (46)
140	64–77 (83)	38–46 (50)
150	68–82 (88)	41–49 (53)
160	73–88 (95)	44–53 (57)
170	77–92 (100)	46–55 (60)
180	82–98 (107)	49–59 (64)
190	86–103 (112)	52–62 (67)
200	91–109 (118)	55–65 (71)

*Healthy body weights are listed on page 85.

We'll begin with the fact that there are about 7 grams of high-quality protein in 1 ounce of cooked meat, poultry, or seafood, ¼ cup of cottage cheese, or 1 egg. Therefore, to meet a high-quality protein goal of, for example, 56 grams, you would need to eat about 8 ounces of meat (8×7 g = 56 g) or the equivalent each day. A typical serving of cooked meat is 3 ounces, about the size of a deck of cards (more at restaurants). You could meet that requirement by having larger-than-average meat servings at two meals a day or eating average servings of meat at at least 3 meals.

In addition to meat, you get high-quality protein—

about 4 grams per serving—from dairy products. A serving equals ½ cup of milk, sour cream, or yogurt, or ⅔ cup of ice cream. Dairy products are restricted in your diet, though, because they contain significant amounts of the several minerals that can cause trouble for people with kidney disease. In general, if your *total* protein requirement is over 100 g per day, you can integrate 2 dairy servings each day; if your requirement is under 100 g per day, limit yourself to 1.

To ensure that you always know how much protein you are getting, we recommend that you weigh the meat portions you eat. Small kitchen balances can be purchased at stores carrying kitchenware. The serving size amounts and grams given here for meat are based on the cooked weight. If you are preparing a mixed dish, you can weigh according to the weight of the raw meat, but you should increase the weight by one-quarter. For instance, if you want 3 ounces cooked you should start with 4 ounces raw. Refer to page 70 for a formula for converting cooked and raw meat weights.

The typical American exceeds the RDA for protein (and calories) daily. On the other hand, people on dialysis very often fail to meet daily protein (and calorie) requirements (though they are the same as the RDA). Most often simple loss of appetite is the reason. Loss of appetite is something that you should discuss with your physician or dietitian as soon as you notice it.

If you do not get enough to eat, you will begin to suffer from a serious condition known as protein wasting. What causes protein wasting is not having the right balance of, or enough, food for a period of time. Your body reacts by burning protein for energy. Protein is available to some extent directly from the food you eat. But when you also don't eat enough protein, your body turns to the protein in your muscles and cells. When protein wasting occurs, your body burns itself up just to get by.

This unhealthy state leads to a spiral of poor health. In particular, protein wasting can cause fatigue and even loss of mental acuity and will make you more susceptible to infections and other acute conditions. The cardinal sign of protein wasting is unintentional weight loss. Sometimes even when you feel like you are eating enough —you feel full or are not hungry—you will begin to lose weight. You need to keep close track of your body weight so that you can be alerted to any problem maintaining weight.

Protein wasting can be prevented by making sure you get enough calories and protein each day. In addition, exercising, even just going for short walks or riding a stationary bike in your home, will serve to stimulate your appetite. Of course, exercise affords many additional health benefits, which we discuss briefly in Chapter Eight.

If you are concerned about or know that you are not getting all the protein you need each day, you can integrate special high-protein powders and mixes into your diet. Protein supplements are available over the counter from many pharmacies, from specialty stores, and through mail order. In the Resources section at the end of this book we provide information on companies that make protein supplements and other diet specialty products. Some will also make available to you recipes that incorporate their products.

Getting enough calories is also a priority. Without enough calories, your body will burn the protein you eat and will not be able to dedicate it to building and repairing muscle and immune cells. There are three general ways to increase the number of calories in your diet. The first is to *eat more food*. With breakfast, eat two pieces of toast and two scrambled eggs instead of one of each. Eat another piece of fruit. Eat a double serving of pot roast (page 107) with your dinner. Have a dessert with lunch and again with dinner. Of course, you don't necessarily want to do this all in the same day, and you do still need to balance your protein intake and restrict certain minerals, but more food is where the calories are. Don't be shy.

The second strategy for increasing your calorie intake is to *add calories to the foods you already eat.* Calorie-enrich foods by adding sweet extras such as jelly, honey, syrup, whipped toppings, and brown sugar; or fat-containing extras such as salad dressings, margarine or butter, mayonnaise, and sour cream. Choose ones with less saturated fat compared to poly- or monounsaturated fats when possible. Be careful not to choose sugar-free (containing artificial sweeteners that have no calories), low-calorie, or "diet" versions of these extras, though. Remember: The point is to increase your calories!

Foods that are easy to dress up include most breads, pastas and rices, salads, and raw and cooked vegetables. Make sure you use plenty of jelly and margarine on your morning toast. Cover the salads and raw vegetables you eat with plenty of your favorite low-sodium dressing; add margarine to fresh cooked vegetables and sugar or nondairy whipped topping to fruit such as sliced peaches or berries. Use plenty of low-sodium mayonnaise (page 95) on your sandwiches and in side salads. Beverages such as fruit juices, ginger ale, and lemonade provide calories—choose them over plain water.

Finally, you can increase calories with certain methods of food preparation. A particularly calorie-dense way to prepare foods is deep-frying. Deep-frying means that the foods are cooked by being submerged in hot oil for a short time. When you fry foods, make sure the batter or other coating is low in sodium, and use liquid vegetable oils such as canola to fry in. (Vegetable oils are lower in saturated fats than animal fats such as fatback or Crisco.) Sautéing is another cooking method where you have the opportunity to add plenty of vegetable oil to the pan when you are cooking meats or vegetables.

Chapter Four

Sodium and Fluid Balance

With the important exception of protein restriction, what is different about the renal diet is the control of micronutrients, food substances that are sprinkled throughout the food you find in the Food Guide Pyramid. **Sodium** is just one of these micronutrients, but it is one of critical importance to people who are concerned about health.

A vast majority of Americans could benefit from reducing the amount of sodium in their diet. High sodium intake is related to many diseases, the most far-reaching of which is high blood pressure, or **hypertension**. Hypertension is directly linked to the development of chronic diseases such as kidney disease and heart disease and is the number one cause of strokes in this country. Since one out of every three Americans is thought to be genetically predisposed to hypertension, it is easy to see that by simply reducing the amount of sodium we consume as a country, the rates of hypertension among our population would drop and the "rate of health" would increase.

Even if you are not predisposed to hypertension (and there is no way to know until symptoms appear), you could benefit from cutting back on sodium, because doing so naturally increases the overall nutritional value of your diet. When you start avoiding processed foods, fast foods, and other salt-laden foods, you will replace them with whole foods. Whole foods are richer sources of all essential nutrients and naturally low in sodium. **Salt, a form of sodium, is the second most common ingredient in processed foods in this country.** Indeed, consuming less sodium will be a major accomplishment on the road to long-term health for our country's population.

As you can imagine, if sodium restriction is so important for healthy individuals in preventing hypertension and kidney disease, it must be imperative for those who already have the disease. This is not easy for many people. The taste for sodium is learned and reinforced over one's lifetime. The level of restriction we recommend for people with kidney disease is not different from levels recommended by the government and other agencies for healthy individuals; yet the absolute importance of sodium restriction does increase in the face of kidney disease. The reason is that sodium restriction is related to improvements in the health of those with kidney disease by helping restore blood pressure and fluid balance to normal levels.

Sodium

Sodium is a chemical element like hydrogen, carbon, and oxygen. It is also called a mineral, which simply indicates that it is a certain type of element. Sodium binds with other elements to form substances we are more familiar with, such as table salt (sodium chloride), baking powder (various sodium compounds), baking soda (sodium bicarbonate), and MSG (monosodium glutamate). These and other high-sodium seasonings and ingredients, such as seasoned salts, preservatives, ketchup, and soy sauce, are common in prepared or processed foods and in recipes. Many are also commonly found on kitchen tables and in restaurants.

Yet sodium is not just a neutral substance you put on your food to make it taste a certain way. The sodium you eat has to be metabolized by your body. The relationship with most sodium molecules is temporary, because your kidneys normally get rid of extra; and the majority of what we eat is extra. The body requires less than 1,000 mg of sodium per day, yet the average person takes in upwards of 8,000 mg per day!

The sodium you do consume enters directly into your blood through your digestive tract. From there it circulates to all your cells, providing them the sodium necessary for proper functioning. Sodium is required for nerve conduction and fluid/electrolyte balance. As blood enters the kidneys, all the extra sodium is aggressively filtered into the urine to be excreted. When kidneys are diseased, sodium excretion is disrupted, and as a result, sodium tends to build up in the blood, where it can cause a lot of trouble. (In some rare types of kidney disease, the kidneys waste sodium instead of retaining it. Whether you are a sodium retainer or a rare salt waster can be determined by your physician.) Whenever sodium balance is disrupted, the body will continually struggle to rebalance its systems.

All kinds of internal mechanisms exist to manage sodium. It is one of the body's goals to keep the concentration of sodium in the blood within a very narrow range. And one way it dilutes the blood is by adding water.

Balancing Fluids

Fluid is lost and fluid is gained. Daily. This happens in everyone. The remarkable thing is we hardly ever even notice.

Fluid is constantly excreted by the body in the form of urine and, to a smaller extent, feces. In addition to these losses, moisture is constantly being formed, and then vaporized away, from your skin and lungs—you can lose three cups or more of fluid each day from vaporization. Internal factors such as activity-induced perspiration, fever, and changes in breathing pattern, and external factors such as temperature and humidity, can influence the amount of water lost through the skin and lungs.

To replace the constant water losses our body experiences, we drink fluids. The solid and semisolid foods we eat also contain a fluid component and therefore contribute to fluid replenishment. A small amount of water is naturally produced by the body during the burning of macronutrients, but it is not enough to make up for what is lost. The body can survive more than 40 days without food, but even a perfectly healthy adult body cannot survive more than 10 days without water.

Balancing the fluid that comes in and the fluid that goes out is something the body does very well. Unfortunately, with the onset of renal disease, this balancing act becomes disrupted and requires special attention.

Sodium and fluid balance are intimately related. Sodium is a water magnet. Because sodium attracts water, the volume of fluid in your blood vessels increases when sodium is high. The body adds water by the activation of your thirst mechanism. By making you thirsty, your body reconstitutes your blood, like a juice drink is reconstituted, according to the sodium it contains. By getting rid of extra sodium, the kidneys keep the body's juice container (its blood vessels) filled to the right capacity. When the kidneys fail in excreting extra sodium, the increased volume of fluid in your blood vessels (the container), in turn, causes your blood pressure to go up. When the extra fluid in your blood vessels forces its way into the surrounding tissues, it causes swelling, or **edema,** in those areas. Edema, which can be painful and crippling, most often occurs in the lower extremities but can also affect organs such as your lungs. This is a common cause of shortness of breath and respiratory distress in people with renal failure.

With fluid accumulated in the blood vessels and tissues, you tend to weigh more. This extra weight is called **water weight** and is different from weight gained because you consume more calories than you need. Water weight gain is characterized by an unusually rapid gain in weight (it can be as much as two pounds in one day) and can cause edema and shortness of breath. The best way to monitor yourself for fluid balance problems is to weigh yourself regularly. You need to have a scale at home so that you can easily keep track of your weight.

When you avoid water weight between dialysis sessions, dialysis is easier. You get less muscle cramping, and, because less fluid has to be removed, there is less strain on your heart, which is sensitive to rapid changes in blood volume. The presence of extra water weight also makes it difficult for your physician and dietitian to know your true body weight. A weight gain of 2 to 5 pounds between each hemodialysis session is reasonable.

In advanced renal failure a person may lose the ability to make adequate amounts of urine. Urine, which is predominantly water, must be passed on a regular basis for normal fluid balance to be maintained. Dialysis can get rid of a fair amount of fluid. Fluid restriction, which is discussed later in this chapter, is especially therapeutic when urine excretion is disrupted.

A state of hypertension develops when there is an overload of fluid and sodium in the blood vessels, and hypertension is a thug that beats up on the kidneys, which are naturally very sensitive to such stressors. It is because of their sensitivity that kidneys are prone to disease in the first place; and that is also why diseased kidneys tend to worsen over time. Yet the *rate* at which your disease worsens is largely under your control.

Restricting Sodium

We recommend for most renal diets a goal of no more than about 2,000 mg of sodium per day. Furthermore, this is the absolute limit for those on hemodialysis. For those on peritoneal dialysis or not on dialysis at all, up to 4,000 mg of sodium per day, and sometimes more, can be *tolerated,* but that does not mean that it is the healthiest level for you. Moreover, if and when you are suffering from edema or heart failure, 2,000 mg should again be your goal. A sodium intake of not over 2,000 or 4,000 mg per day will help keep your kidneys and your body under a minimum amount of stress.

A very small percentage of people with renal disease actually have to supplement sodium in their diet because their kidneys waste sodium rather than retain it. Specifically, people with interstitial nephritis, which is most often related to pyelonephritis, drug nephropathy, or polycystic kidney disease, are prone to be sodium excreters rather than sodium retainers and to have low blood pressure rather than high. Only a physician can determine this; medications treat the condition.

The vast majority of people with kidney failure retain the sodium they eat. For all but those mentioned above, radically reducing the amount of dietary sodium *will* have an undeniably positive effect. You'll feel better all around.

The most common form of sodium used today is table salt. The first step to sodium restriction is putting down the salt shaker. Many other common seasonings contain significant amounts of sodium.

Some High-Sodium Seasonings to Eliminate (mg sodium in 1 teaspoon)
Table salt (2,130)　"Lite" salt (1,100)　Soy sauce (343) Seasoned salts—garlic salt, celery salt, etc. (1,600) Meat tenderizer (1,750) MSG, Accent (500)

Some High-Sodium Seasonings to Use Moderately (mg sodium in 1 teaspoon)
Ketchup (67)　Mustard (65)　Worcestershire sauce (49) Chili, barbecue, or steak sauces (80)　Pickle relish (35) Parmesan cheese (31)

If you check the labels on these seasonings and many others, you can see the prominent role sodium has in their composition. Seasonings high in sodium need to be either eliminated or used in great moderation if you want to achieve your low-sodium goal.

The high-sodium seasonings we recommend you eliminate, such as those in the top half of the table above, are those that are salty for salty's sake. They have very little purpose other than to imbue food with a salty flavor. Seasonings in the lower half of table, the moderate-use category, have other nutrients in them and can be used occasionally in relatively small amounts in cooking or preparing meals.

Because sodium is a chemical part of many additives and preservatives, it is present in many processed foods. The taste of sodium is obvious in some foods but not in others. For example, many cereals and breads, enriched or not, contain sodium-bound minerals or sodium-based leaveners such as baking soda or baking powder. Because starches are the basis of your diet, it is important that you find brands and types of cereals and breads that are lowest in sodium. Don't just assume that all similar products are the same nutritionally. **Remember: Always check the label for sodium, because foods don't have to taste salty to contain lots of sodium.**

Other processed foods, such as microwave dinners, canned meats and vegetables, and flavor packets and dinner mixes, are almost guaranteed to have more sodium added as seasonings and preservatives than you need. Do not buy these kinds of foods unless you are certain they have been specially designed to be low in sodium.

As a strategy for keeping your sodium within the goal of 2,000 mg per day, we recommend that, in general, no one item you eat exceed 250 mg of sodium. In terms of nutrition labels, it is important that you consider the serving size of an item. You need to acknowledge how much of the food you will eat and, therefore, how much sodium you will be getting from it at one time.

Some nonprescription drugs, such as cough syrup and Alka-Seltzer, also contain large amounts of sodium. Check with your physician or pharmacist about alternative low-sodium medications.

There is a danger in today's rapidly changing food market of overgeneralizing and overrestricting based on the way things used to be. Foods that have (and always will contain) lots of sodium are regular hard cheeses, deli

Sodium-related claims that can appear on food labels:

- *Sodium-free or salt-free.* Less than 5 mg of sodium *per serving;* the sodium content is acceptable, but what else does it contain?
- *Very low sodium.* Less than 35 mg of sodium *per serving;* again, the sodium content is acceptable, but what else does it contain?
- *Low-sodium.* Less than 140 mg *per serving, per 2 tablespoons,* or *per 50 g,* whichever is greater; the sodium content for one serving is acceptable, so watch out how much of it you eat.
- *Light in sodium.* There is a reduction in sodium of 50 percent or less *compared to the content of a reference food;* this is not a guarantee that it contains an acceptable amount of sodium.
- *Reduced or less sodium.* There is a reduction in sodium of 25 percent or less *compared to the content of a reference food;* again, this is not a guarantee that it contains an acceptable amount of sodium.
- *No salt added, unsalted, or without added salt.* No *salt* was added during processing; this does not mean it is low in sodium, since sodium comes in many forms other than salt.

or cured meats, fast foods, and canned or restaurant soups. Yet today there are low-sodium cheeses, meats, and soups available in grocery and specialty stores, in catalogs, and on restaurant menus. This trend is definitely positive, but we recommend that you continue to: (1) focus on your overall dietary needs rather than be drawn in by fancy claims and (2) be a smart consumer by asking,

There Are 1,000 mg of Sodium in This Much of These . . .

High-sodium foods	Low-sodium foods
½ t table salt	500 T of herb mixture
1 specialty hamburger (fast food)	11 svgs. of Peas-&-Potato Mash (see p. 125)
1 enchilada (fast food)	7 plain beef tacos (fast food)
10 green olives	6 lbs of carrots
2 slices of commercial cheese pizza	18 Vegetable Calzones (see p. 113)
1 bacon and egg breakfast sandwich (fast food)	24 bowls of shredded wheat cereal and milk
7 c of sport beverage	25 c of ginger ale
3 oz of cooked ham	40 oz of plain, cooked fish
1 c of canned soup	20 c Dill Tuna-Noodle Chowder (see p. 93)
3 apple pies (fast food)	12 c vanilla ice cream
1 large dill pickle	1,000 apples
2 large pieces of cornbread	7 slices of regular white bread

"In taking out the salt, have they added something else that is not good for me?" A good example of this phenomenon is salt substitutes. In salt substitutes, sodium is simply replaced by potassium, another mineral that is restricted in renal diets. (Salt substitutes are also harmful because they work by tricking your taste buds into thinking you are still eating salt, making it more difficult to stop eating salty food.) If you have questions about whether certain reformulated products fit into the renal diet, you can always call the manufacturer for more information or talk to a registered dietitian.

Learning to Love Low-Sodium Food

It takes the taste buds approximately six weeks to adjust to and begin liking the taste of reduced-salt foods. Our affinity for very salty foods is thought to be an innate mechanism that developed to ensure adequate intake during times when salt was not readily available and activity, which increases salt losses, was more intense. Today, people are living longer and longer lives, and chronic diseases such as hypertension, kidney disease, and heart disease are the most serious threat to health. Of course, salt is readily available, and people are less active than ever before. It is no longer need that drives our sodium consumption but habit. By our history, it is easy to see why sodium is so readily habit forming; in time, though, you won't miss it.

In addition to time, you need creativity and an open mind to enjoy low-sodium food. You must learn to appreciate the more subtle, natural flavors of food and combine ingredients in tasty ways so that flavor is best enhanced. Sodium is found naturally in small amounts in whole foods but never in the amounts typically consumed by salt-happy Americans. Until now, many of us have unwittingly allowed our innate liking of sodium to substitute for creativity in preparing food.

One way to learn about and try different food combinations is to try good recipes. The last chapter of this book contains 45 recipes low in sodium and generally suited to a renal diet. There are many other cookbooks and recipe sources out there. After the recipe chapter you will find a Resources section and a Further Reading section; the latter includes the names of cookbooks, and remember, don't be afraid to alter the ingredients a little to suit your tastes (see page 65 for how to adapt recipes). No recipe is set in stone. The point is to broaden your options.

One of the most important factors in creative low-salt cooking is the use of herbs and spices. In general, herbs are thought of as the leaves of aromatic plants whereas spices are the (usually ground) roots or seeds of such plants. Though each of us has his or her own personal tastes, certain combinations of foods with herbs and spices are naturally enhancing. We have included a detailed description of common herbs and spices and their best uses in Appendix A. Herbs and spices can make (or occasionally break) a dish, so the first rule in experimental cooking is to add them a little bit at a time. Start with one-quarter of a teaspoon or less of each dry herb or spice for every 4 servings (depending on how many different herbs and spices you will add; start with 1 or 2 at a time). For fresh herbs, use up to three times the amount as for dry, and in recipes triple the amount if given for dry herb. Any finely ground spice or herb will impart its flavor more quickly than do leaves or seeds, so add leaves and seeds more toward the beginning of cooking and ground spices more toward the end.

Be creative with the foods you are used to eating. For instance, a good-tasting alternative to a plain old ground beef patty can be made by crumbling a cooked ground beef patty into several ounces of cooked macaroni, and adding your favorite low-sodium flavorings, such as thyme, Tabasco sauce, or a dash of vinegar for a kick, and a pat of unsalted margarine. With or without a recipe to guide you, you can create many satisfying foods with just a little imagination.

In general, hot spices such as chili powder and cayenne pepper can wake up just about any food. But to give foods a kick without making yourself sweat, dash a little vinegar or lemon juice on what you are making. These tangy additions will literally make your mouth water and will accentuate the natural flavors of the food. If you avoid certain vegetables because they have a bitter taste, try adding a dash of sugar (white or brown) to neutralize the bitterness.

Fluid Restriction and Thirst

In terms of dietary changes, we emphasize the strict moderation of sodium rather than fluid restriction. This is because when sodium is restricted, fluid naturally restricts itself. If you do not overdo it with sodium, you will not drink too much fluid. Indeed, though, if your urine output decreases because of your kidney disease, it becomes necessary that you consciously limit the amount of fluid you take in.

Drinking copious amounts of water is often recommended for attaining good health, but that changes when the kidneys stop producing enough urine. Like turning down the heat on a pot of water that is boiling over, you must turn down the amount of fluid you take in, or fluid will pour over into your tissues, raising your blood pressure, and causing water weight gain and edema. Such problems are indications that you are taking in too much sodium and fluid. To help your body maintain a proper fluid balance, *use thirst as your guide.*

For a person on hemodialysis whose urine output has decreased, a rough guideline for fluid restriction is urine output (yes, you should measure that) plus 700 mL (3 cups). Keep weight gains between dialysis sessions to less than five pounds. Weigh yourself daily to monitor this. When you see you are gaining weight rapidly, reduce your fluid intake—and especially your sodium intake—further.

As much as 2,000 mL (8-½ cups) *total* can be tolerated by those on peritoneal dialysis. For those not on dialysis, fluid is not restricted until urine output decreases. Any time you notice a sustained decrease in your urine output, make an appointment to see your physician.

The definition of a fluid is anything that is liquid at room temperature. This includes all beverages, ice, frozen desserts, and gelatin but does not include liquid fats such as oils. There are certain fluids that should be avoided by anyone with renal disease: cola drinks, Tang, and sports drinks. This is because they contain minerals that should be restricted. Everyone should limit the amounts of coffee, tea, and alcohol they drink; more nourishing beverages include juice and milk.

Here are some easy ways to avoid drinking excessive amounts of fluid:

- Drink only when you are thirsty and drink only enough to satisfy your thirst.
- Drink from very small cups or glasses.
- Take your medications with mealtime beverages to reduce the need for more fluids later.
- Do not drink simply from habit or to be social. You can stand without a glass in your hand at a party and no one will notice!

If you find yourself suffering a dry mouth and know you are pushing your fluid restriction limit, there are some techniques you can use to relieve thirst, at least temporarily. Try sucking on some hard sour candies, an ice cube, or a lemon wedge, or chewing gum to stimulate saliva in your mouth. Try rinsing your mouth with water. Eat a piece of cold fruit—some people even like to suck on frozen grapes. Most important, though, try even harder to minimize the amount of sodium you are eating.

Chapter Five

Potassium and Phosphorus

Potassium

The mineral potassium is found in fruits and vegetables, nuts and dry beans, dairy products and meats. There is very little in bread, pasta, and rice, and none in oil, butter, and margarine. Most of the potassium a person takes in comes from fruits and vegetables. Certain fruits and vegetables contain very high amounts, while others contain significantly less.

Once absorbed into the blood by the gut, instead of being concentrated in our blood like sodium, potassium is concentrated in our body's cells, where it is required for nerve conduction and muscle contraction.

When a cell has enough potassium, it sends extra into the blood, where it circulates around to be taken up by other cells that might need it. Potassium in the blood is extra. Ten to 15 percent of the potassium in your blood is normally excreted into the urine. Thus the kidneys "act" on potassium by simply leaking a certain amount of it. Nothing more complicated than that. Like a small hole at the bottom of a barrel full of water, potassium trickles slowly but steadily out of normally functioning kidneys to be eliminated by the body.

With renal failure the potassium leak stops up. Since we are constantly taking in potassium through what we eat, our body begins to "overflow" with potassium. And too much is dangerous.

Potassium is particularly important for proper nerve conduction. Therefore, accumulate too much and the nerve cells that are most sensitive, those in the heart, get overstimulated. Since your heart relies on the periodic, potassium-regulated electrical stimulation of the heart muscles to beat, potassium overload endangers the integrity of your heartbeat. It can cause the heart to start beating erratically, or to slow to a stop. These life-threatening situations *most often arise suddenly and without warning.* This is one reason all patients on dialysis are required to have monthly "chemistries," blood tests that measure the levels of potassium and other minerals. Such tests can reveal potential problems developing with your potassium level and, thus, are important in preventing complications involving the heart.

Some people are more prone to potassium overload and its complications because of the particular condition affecting their kidneys. For instance, diabetes mellitus and chronic urinary tract obstruction cause a kind of kidney disease that is accompanied by alterations in potassium excretion, whereas most renal disease does not affect potassium regulation until <20 percent of renal function remains.

The potassium restriction guidelines given here are based on the typical person with advanced renal failure and are fairly strict. Though some people could "get away" with less restriction, we highly recommend that you aim to meet the guidelines. It will not harm you to be cautious about potassium and can only be good for your kidneys and your heart.

Managing Potassium

For those not on dialysis, potassium is not usually restricted until a measure of kidney function called glomerular filtration rate (GFR)—a measure similar to creatinine clearance—shows considerable decline. Your physician should talk to you about this measurement. It is a good idea to ask about potassium restriction so that your physician will know that you want to be informed when it is necessary. At that point, a consultation with a dietitian would be helpful since a dietitian can give you advice based on your specific circumstances and answer specific questions you may have.

Because potassium is not itself a macronutrient like protein and you don't add it to foods for flavor like sodium, potassium is easier to monitor and vary without disrupting the rest of your diet. One simple way to monitor your potassium intake, and the way we recommend, is to categorize fruits and vegetables according to the amount of potassium in a typical serving. In the tables on pages 53 and 54 we have divided fruits and vegetables into three groups—those containing low, moderate, and high levels of potassium.

While potatoes are in the high-potassium group, one option is to leach some of the potassium away before eating them. Peel them, slice them thin or grate them, and soak them overnight in water before cooking. Much of the potassium leaves the food and goes into the water.

If you are using leached potatoes consider them in the moderate potassium group.

The way to limit potassium in the renal diet is to limit the number of high-potassium fruits and vegetables you

Category of Potassium Content for Select Vegetables

(Serving equals ½ cup cooked unless stated otherwise)

Low potassium: Less than 125 mg per serving	Moderate potassium: 125–225 mg per serving	High potassium: More than 225 mg per serving
Cabbage	Asparagus	Lima beans
Cucumber	Broccoli	Potatoes
Green beans	Beets	Spinach
Iceberg lettuce (1 cup)	Carrots	Tomatoes
Mushrooms (½ cup raw, sliced)	Corn	Vegetable juices such as carrot
Bell peppers	Eggplant	Winter squash*
	Green peas	
	Looseleaf lettuce (1 cup)	
	Onion	
	Zucchini and other summer squash	

*Off the scale; do not eat

eat. In general, think of choosing mostly low-potassium items, selectively choosing some moderate-potassium items, and, depending on the severity of your restriction, avoiding high-potassium items. If you effectively restrict potassium, you will greatly reduce your risk of sudden heart failure and to some extent relieve symptoms such as muscle weakness and fatigue. In general, controlling potassium will be harder for big eaters because they are restricted to the same absolute amount of potassium but eat more food. Big eaters need to focus even more on eating the lowest-potassium fruits and vegetables.

After glancing over the lists of fruits and vegetables,

Category of Potassium Content for Select Fruits

(Serving equals ½ cup raw unless stated otherwise)

Low potassium: Less than 100 mg per serving	Moderate potassium: 100–200 mg per serving	High potassium: More than 200 mg per serving
Apple (1 small)	Apple juice	Apricots (3 ea.)
Blueberries	Blackberries	Avocado*
Fruit cocktail, canned	Grapefruit (½ ea.) Peach (1 ea.)	Banana (1 ea.) Cantaloupe
Cranberries	Sweet cherries (10 ea.)	Kiwi fruit (1 ea.)
Cranberry juice	Pears (1 ea.)	Honeydew melon
Grapes (10 ea.)	Pineapple, canned	Orange (1 ea.)
Mandarin oranges, canned	Raisins (2 tablespoons) Raspberries	Orange juice Prunes*
Peaches, canned	Strawberries	
Pineapple, fresh	Tangerine (1 ea.)	
Plum (1 large)	Watermelon (1 cup)	

*Off the scale; do not eat

you probably almost immediately discovered that there is at least one fruit or vegetable you want to know about that is not listed. This brings up a particular difficulty you will face in monitoring your potassium. Unlike sodium content, potassium content is not required to be published and so is rarely included on manufacturer's food nutrition labels. In addition, if you buy fresh fruits and vegetables they have no labels at all. But that does not put the information beyond your reach. Many grocery stores now provide a fairly complete nutritional analysis alongside produce items. You can use these nutritional analyses to decide right then and there which items are best for you to buy. Take a pen and paper with you to the store and jot down the potassium, protein, and phosphorus content of the produce you buy so you can have that information at home.

Sooner or later you will want to do your own research. You can get comprehensive food nutrient tables from a dietitian or health advocacy group at your workplace or nearby medical center. National organizations such as the National Kidney Foundation also distribute such tables. In our Resources section you will find a listing of national organizations offering such literature and services.

There are other sources of potassium besides fruits and vegetables. It is no further loss to eliminate nuts and dry beans, since those should be eliminated based on their low-quality protein content anyway. Dairy products and meats both contain a fair amount of potassium. In general, dairy products are limited in the renal diet in part because of the potassium and phosphorus they contain. The potassium and phosphorus in meat, on the other hand, is tolerated in the renal diet. Meats are included because of their high-quality protein; the potassium they contain is corrected for by the limits on high-potassium fruits and vegetables.

Exactly how much potassium can I have? For people on hemodialysis we recommend that your potassium intake be restricted to between 2,000 and 3,000 mg per day; for those on peritoneal dialysis or with general renal insufficiency requiring potassium restriction, to between 3,000 and 4,000 mg per day. Monitor potassium in the same way you do the other nutrients you eat; keep a running daily tally. Pat yourself on the back every time you are able to keep your potassium low for the day.

Phosphorus

Phosphorus is found in large amounts in high-protein foods like meats, dairy products, nuts, and dry beans, as well as in cola drinks, beer, and chocolate (in particular, cocoa). Because it is a common ingredient in many preservatives, it is also abundant in processed foods such as breakfast foods (dry cereals, instant hot cereals). (Note: For some reason, *quick* hot cereals are better than instant.)

Most people's diets contain significantly more phosphorus than their body needs. The digestive system allows as much as 30 percent of the phosphorus eaten to be passed into the stool. Still, what we absorb is a significant amount. The body puts phosphorus to use in maintaining strong teeth and bones and in making DNA and energy molecules in the cells. There is a paradox attached to phosphorus, though. Too much of it disrupts the same things for which it is useful, particularly the bones.

Too much phosphorus is usually not a critical problem for people whose kidneys are fully functioning, though it is thought to contribute to the long-term development of osteoporosis (a disease where the bones become thin and brittle) and joint degeneration in many people. **Renal bone disease** is the name of the condition that develops quite rapidly once phosphorus levels become very high in individuals with kidney disease. Renal bone disease is similar to osteoporosis except that its symptoms are more acute and its cause and treatment different.

Many people think only of calcium, another mineral responsible for bone health, when they think of bone diseases. Indeed, having enough calcium in your diet is essential for strong bones. Yet too much phosphorus can undermine bone health as much as too little calcium. When phosphorus, which is normally excreted by the kidneys, begins to build up in the blood, calcium, which is the primary mineral in bone, is drawn from the bone into the blood because of its strong affinity for phosphorus. And calcium cannot benefit the skeleton when it is in the blood. Phosphorus-mediated decalcification of the bones is the cause of renal bone disease.

Symptoms of renal bone disease include bone and joint pain and muscle weakness. It can also present very dramatically and seriously with a bone fracture, or more subtly and annoyingly with itchiness. Itchiness is an important barometer of phosphorus overload in some, a warning sign that, if heeded, can keep bone disease from developing further.

Managing Phosphorus

Science has had success in helping control phosphorus blood levels in kidney disease. It has been known for some time that certain substances, when taken with high-phosphorus foods, seem to interfere with the absorption of phosphorus from the intestine. These substances, which have come to be known as **phosphorus binders,** are essential in preventing renal bone disease.

Your doctor will prescribe a certain amount of phosphorus binder to take with meals. The amount of phosphorus in your diet is closely related to the amount of protein, so your prescription is based largely on your protein requirement. There are different types and forms of binder medication. Calcium carbonate, which is an antacid available over the counter, and calcium acetate are common types and should be taken according to your doctor's orders. Binders most often come as tablets, chewable or otherwise.

Here are some hints on getting the most from your phosphorus binders:

- Take binder during your meal or immediately before or after (within 10 minutes).
- Larger than ordinary meals usually require more binder.
- To reduce the number of pills you have to take, add crushed binder pills to food such as applesauce, mashed potatoes, and baked goods.
- Don't forget to take your binder with you when you go out to eat.
- Some people experience constipation as a result of taking phosphorus binders. If this becomes a problem for you, ask your doctor about stool softeners that can be taken in conjunction with binders.

The best approach to restricting the phosphorus in your diet is to follow your protein guidelines for meat and dairy product consumption. Another thing you can do is eliminate high-phosphorus beverages such as colas and beer. A few foods that you wouldn't necessarily expect to be high in phosphorus but are include frozen yogurt and dark rye bread. Just be aware.

Chapter Six

Meal Planning

W hat do you say to yourself when your stomach starts to grumble or your energy level decreases? Probably "I'm hungry" or "I'd better eat something." As infants, we met this need by crying; as adults, we engage in meal planning. Meal planning is making decisions about what, when, where, how, and with whom to eat. We will focus only on the what-to-eat of meal planning.

Making Choices

There are six food-choice categories that the renal diet centers on. They correspond to the six food groups in the Food Guide Pyramids (see pages 12 and 13). We will refer to the groups simply as Starch, Vegetable, Fruit, Meat, Dairy, and Fat. The number of items from each group that you should eat each day depends on your activity level, calorie requirements, and weight-loss status, but the proportions among the groups are constant. General guidelines to these proportions, given as a range of number of servings in the various groups, can be found in the Food Guide Pyramids. On page 61 is a table that lists foods that fit into each category, the amount that counts

as one serving, as well as that category's nutritional definition—approximately how much of each nutrient that
type of food contains.

Because of space limitations, the table only includes a
fraction of the foods that are actually available to you. Determine how well a food not contained in the table fits into
your diet by comparing the information on its label with
the numbers in this table, which are only general guidelines. Few foods will correspond exactly to these guidelines—that is the nature of food variety—but there are
always some foods in each group that fit better than others.

The table also defines a single serving size amount for
the food items listed. As with nutrition labels, serving
size—or, rather, how much you *will* eat—is something
that you must consider when choosing foods and planning your meals. For example, you may be surprised to
hear that 1 cup (8 ounces) of milk—an amount that
some automatically consider a single serving—actually
counts as 2 dairy servings. So if you drink 1 cup of milk
you will be getting twice the protein, calories, phosphorus, etc., listed under 1 serving. One cup of milk *can* be
appropriate, but only if you are aware of the fact that you
are getting 2 servings of dairy.

To avoid confusion about how much food you are
eating, we encourage you to prepare or serve up all your
snacks and meals in their entirety before you start eating.
If you are eating out, take a survey of all the food you
have, decide how much of each item you will eat, and
make a mental note of what you eat so you can accurately
record it later. Another way to educate yourself about
serving sizes is to take a look at measuring cups and
spoons. Just how much is one half of a cup, anyway?

There is perhaps still some question as to *what* foods
to include or not include in your diet. Many recommendations have been made throughout chapters Three,
Four, and Five. For example, do not eat dried beans and

Foods, Serving Sizes, and Nutritional Definitions for Each Renal Diet Choice

Starch
1 slice of white bread
⅔ c cooked rice
½ c pasta
2 graham crackers
5 unsalted crackers
1 small slice of cake/pie
½ c hot cereal
¾ c cold cereal
1 c unsalted popcorn
4 butter cookies
1 sweet roll

Fruit
1 apple, peach, small pear, orange, or tangerine
½ grapefruit
1 c watermelon pieces
3 plums
2 T raisins
20 grapes
10 cherries
½ c applesauce, berries, fruit cocktail, pineapple, or fruit juice

Vegetable
½ c cooked
¾ c raw

Meat
1 egg
1 oz cooked boneless meat or fish
⅓ of a chicken or turkey breast or large pork chop
5 shrimp or oysters
¼ c cottage cheese

Dairy
½ c milk or half & half
⅔ c ice cream or frozen yogurt
½ c sour cream
½ c yogurt, any type

Fat
1 t oil or butter
1 T salad dressing or mayonnaise

Amount in one serving	Starch	Fruit	Vegetable	Meat	Dairy	Fat
Calories	70	80	35	75	varies	45
HQ protein	0 g	0 g	1–2 g*	7 g	4 g	0 g
LQ protein	2 g	0.5 g		0 g	0 g	0 g
Sodium**	130 mg	2 mg	10 mg	25 mg	60 mg	0–50 mg
Potassium	30 mg	200 mg***	200 mg***	100 mg	175 mg	0 g
Phosphorus	25 mg	15 mg	40 mg	70 mg	115 mg	0 g

* See the table on page 25 for a list of vegetables with higher protein.
** Choosing low-sodium brands can reduce this amount.
*** Varies; see the tables on pages 53 and 54 for categories of potassium content.

peas because of their low-quality protein; avoid cheeses because they tend to be high in sodium and phosphorus. It is not helpful to overgeneralize about food, though. The food market is changing every day; moreover, it seems there are always exceptions to food rules. So instead of making additional lists of foods to eat and foods to avoid, we will phrase your food choices in terms of the restrictions you already know.

General Criteria for Choosing Foods According to Food Group	
Group	Watch Out For . . .
Starch	protein (low-quality) and sodium
Vegetable	potassium, sodium if canned, and, to a small extent, protein
Fruit	potassium, fluids if fruit juices
Meat	amount consumed (weighing portions is recommended); sodium (specifically deli meats); requires phosphorus binder
Dairy	amount and type consumed; sodium (specifically cheeses); requires phosphorus binder
Fat	type (minimize saturated fats); amount

The table above applies the various nutrient restrictions covered in the last three chapters to your food choices. It identifies what nutrients in each food group to focus your restriction on. An example of how this kind of thinking can help in making food decisions is that you know you need not worry about protein when choosing a fruit to eat—concentrate on potassium content.

See your diet as a series of choices about what to eat and not as an overall restriction. It is not realistic to think in terms of restricting every food for every nutrient or evaluating every possible food for every potential positive and negative. You have to eat—this is not a starvation diet! The point is not to stop enjoying eating but to start eating in a way that is right for your kidneys.

Another Word About Diabetes

Fortunately, for those of you already familiar with the diabetic exchanges diet, the renal meal planning guidelines presented here are not radically different. What we refer to as choices are essentially the same thing as exchanges in the diabetic diet. In fact, a different word was chosen for the simple reason that otherwise the two regimens might easily be confused with each other.

What is different, and more difficult, for those who must also follow the dietary guidelines for diabetes is that there are more restrictions to consider when choosing foods. The good thing is that you have most likely been following the diabetic diet for a long time now, so you have that base to work from. If you are concerned about your food choices being too limited, it is time to go in search of new foods you have not yet explored. For instance, you may have snacked mostly on salt-free nuts, which are not recommended on a renal diet. Other crunchy snack foods—which are also low in sugar, salt, *and* low-quality protein—include low-sodium cereals such as corn and wheat squares. In Chapter Nine you will find a recipe for a snack mix that is a smart snack for the renal and diabetes combination diet.

Balancing Your Choices Daily

Like deciding which roads to take when driving or what time to go to bed and then wake up, choosing what to eat means continual decision making. When following a diet, there are no perfectly correct decisions, only better or worse ones.

We have so far been focusing on making individual food choices; we will now turn to how to get the proper balance of foods each day. Only a complete diet can provide you with all the nutrients you require. And eating according to the six food categories will help you to cover those requirements. In the Food Guide Pyramids on pages 12 and 13 there are ranges for the number of items to eat. The table below gives a more specific guideline of how to balance the food groups given the constraints of the renal diet. The balance reflected in this table is based on protein requirement only. Other factors influence your dietary needs, so recommendations for your particular case are best determined by a dietitian familiar with your habits, requirements, and lifestyle.

Number of Daily Choices According to Total Protein Requirement (p. 28 or p. 32)							
Prescribed protein intake	40 g	50 g	60 g	70 g	80 g	90 g	100 g
Starch*	4	5	6	7	8	9	9
Vegetable*	3	3	4	4	4	5	5
Fruit	4	4	4	4	4	4	4
Meat	3	4	5	6	7	8	9
Dairy	1	1	1	1	1	1	2
Fat	5	5	5	6	6	6	6
Average Calories Provided	1,230	1,375	1,555	1,745	1,890	2,070	2,220

* Make use of low-protein flour/breads and avoid higher-protein vegetables (p. 25) to increase the number of choices in these categories.

The calories provided by the diet outlined for the lowest protein levels are moderately low. What do we recommend if your calorie requirement (see page 19) exceeds the average provided by the foods you can fit in your diet? To increase calories without exceeding your protein level, make use of more low-protein breads, pastas, and flours. On the other hand, if you are considering losing weight, you will need to aim at reducing your calorie intake anyway, so you may not want to add any more calories. Keep in mind, though, that we do not recommend that anyone eat fewer than 1,200 calories per day on a regular basis without the guidance of a dietitian.

If you are on dialysis or for some other reason need to keep weight on, you have to be sure to get enough calories each day. Eat high-calorie versions of some foods. For example, you could eat 1 serving of ice cream instead of drinking a serving of skim milk for your dairy choice. Additional calories should be added as low-potassium fruits or fruit juices, fats, and sweets. This is because, in general, all of the food choices except fat and fruits (and sweets are comparable to fruit) contain protein, and protein has to be carefully balanced.

Fats can be added as butter or margarine, low-sodium salad dressings, and mayonnaise. Examples of sweets that are good are hard candies, gum drops, butter mints, honey, maple syrup (no molasses, though), and lemon bars. Avoid chocolate as it contains a lot of phosphorus. Cakes, cookies, and fruit-based pies are often good choices for adding calories. Remember to avoid desserts containing nuts. There is more on protein wasting and increasing calorie intake on pages 33–35.

Adapting Recipes

A recipe is a specified way of making or doing something. Food recipes usually include a list of ingredients and directions on how to combine the ingredients into a finished

Sample Food Record for a Moderately Active (150-lb) Person with Renal Insufficiency

Food Items	Number of choices				
	Starch	Veget.	Fruit	Meat (1 oz)	Dairy
GOAL	5	3	4	4	1
1 egg scrambled				1	
1 pc mixed grain bread	1				
1½ t unsalted margarine					
1 c coffee w/sugar & nondairy creamer					
½ c orange juice			1		
1 salad (1 c lettuce, ½ c veg.)		1			
1 t grated Parmesan cheese					0.5
2 T vinaigrette dressing (p. 95)					
1 baked potato, flesh only	1				
¼ c reduced fat sour cream					0.5
1 peach w/nondairy topping			1		
1 c ginger ale					
3 oz East Indian Sautéed Chicken (p. 108)				3	
1 svg. Saffron Rice (p. 130)	1				
½ c fresh cooked carrots		1			
½ c fresh cooked spinach		1			
2 t unsalted margarine					
1 c lemon-lime soda					
1 pc Blueberry Cake (p. 139)	1		1		
½ c cranberry-apple juice			1		
2 graham crackers	1				
TOTAL	5	3	4	4	1

There is a blank copy of this form in Appendix B. Use it in record keeping.

| | | *Amount* | | |
Fat (1 t)	Extra calories	Protein (g)	High-quality?	Sodium (mg)
5	var.	50	<30	<2,000
		7	7	65
		2.5		125
1.5				
	X			10
		1		
		0.5		
		1	1	40
1				10
		3		10
		2	2	25
	X	0.5		
	X			20
		21	21	55
0.5		3		30
		1		
		2		20
2				
	X			30
		3.5		115
		2		85
5		50	31	640

Sample Food Record for a Moderately Active (150-lb) Person on Hemodialysis

Food Items	Number of choices				
	Starch	Veget.	Fruit	Meat (1 oz)	Dairy
GOAL	9	5	4	7	1
1 egg				1	
½ c gr. pepper & onion		0.5			
1 pc toast—white	1				
1 t unsalted margarine					
1 t jam					
½ grapefruit			1		
3 oz cooked skinless chicken breast				3	
1 sandwich bun	2				
1 T homemade mayonnaise (p. 94)					
1 c carrot sticks		1			
½ c lemonade					
3 peach halves, canned in juice			1		
⅔ c low-fat vanilla ice cream					1
1 medium apple			1		
3 oz Pot Roast + veg. (p. 106)		0.5		3	
1 svg. Mushroom & Rice Cass. (p. 119)	2	0.5			
1 c fresh cooked green beans		2			
1 t margarine					
1 pc lemon pie	1		1		
1 English muffin	2				
2 T apple butter					
2 graham crackers	1				
TOTAL	9	4.5	4	7	1

There is a blank copy of this form in Appendix B. Use it in record keeping.

Fat (1 t)	Extra calories	Amount Protein (g)	High-quality?	Sodium (mg)
6	var.	82	>50	<2,000
		7	7	65
		1		
		2		165
1				
	X			10
		0.5		
		21	21	50
		4		250
1.5				
	X			
		1		10
0.5		4	4	160
		0.5		
0.5		24	21	65
		4		60
		3		
1				
1.5		4		130
		4		250
	X			
		2		85
6		82	53	1,300

product. We encourage you to alter any of the details of a recipe to make it meet your special dietary needs and to make the food taste good to you. Recipes are essential to meal planning, so use them. Basically, successfully adapting recipes for the renal diet means manipulating sources of protein, sodium, and to some extent potassium.

To begin, identify sources of these nutrients in a recipe. Meats, eggs, dairy products, nuts, dried beans, and peas will contribute significant amounts of protein. We recommend you greatly limit nuts, dried beans, and peas, so instead try: (1) substituting a vegetable like green peas; (2) reducing the amount called for in the recipe; or (3) just leaving the ingredient out—it probably will not be missed if there is a variety of other ingredients in the recipe. We do not recommend leaving out or making substitutions for eggs. There are 7 grams of high-quality protein in one egg, and egg protein is the best of all. So use the recipe, with the eggs, and just count the protein it contributes in your daily total.

Another strategy is to alter the amount of meat in a recipe when necessary. Remember: Protein grams are counted according to the cooked weight of the meat, so when looking at a recipe that calls for a certain amount of raw meat, you will need to be able to estimate the amount of cooked meat and the serving sizes that the recipe will yield. Use the following formula to make such conversions:

Amount in each cooked serving = amt of raw meat to begin with ÷# servings x 0.75 (cooking factor);

Amount of raw meat to begin with = # servings x cooked serving size x 1.25 (cooking factor).

Remember: 1 ounce of **cooked** meat = 7 grams of high-quality protein;

1 pound of **raw** meat = 16 ounces of raw meat but 12 ounces of cooked meat.

To determine the approximate size of each serving of cooked meat that will result from the amount of raw meat called for in the recipe, use the first equation. To change the amount of raw meat you begin with—for example, if you do not want to make as many servings as are produced by the recipe, or if you want to make the servings smaller in size—use the second equation. (The math is relatively simple, but a calculator or adding machine is helpful.) The elements of each equation can be switched around to determine the other variables.

Dairy products are another high-protein, high-phosphorus and sometimes high-sodium ingredient in recipes. Cheeses that are high in sodium should be eliminated from recipes and, if necessary, lower-sodium alternatives substituted. In addition to many natural cheeses, nearly all processed cheeses or cheese spreads are high in sodium. For example, 1 ounce of processed American cheese contains 406 mg of sodium. Some cheeses that naturally contain less than 150 mg of sodium per ounce include cream cheese, mozzarella, Swiss, Gruyère, and Neufchâtel. In addition, lower-sodium versions of some high-sodium cheeses are now available. Remember to count the protein from dairy products (see the table on page 61).

Another workable substitution for dairy products is nondairy creamer for milk. Nondairy creamers are available in the dairy cases of many grocery stores. They are low in phosphorus, sodium, and protein. They do, on the other hand, contain more potassium—as much as a moderate-potassium vegetable—than dairy products, so consider that in your meal planning. Use them as an alternative to milk in recipes where milk is used as a nonbaking liquid, such as in soups and rice casseroles. They are not recommended as a direct substitute in baked goods.

The next step in adapting recipes is to look more closely at the sodium and potassium they contain. We already discussed low-sodium cheese substitutions. In addition to salty food ingredients, table salt is often added to recipes by default and therefore is not missed when it is left out or used in a reduced amount. For example, cooking directions for pastas and rices often call for adding salt to the cooking water. In this and most all other similar situations, the salt is not necessary—just leave it out. When you look at a recipe and see that it calls for salt, ask yourself, Will this dish—pan-fried fish or French toast or pot roast or zucchini quiche—taste all right without the ½ teaspoon of salt it calls for? Usually the answer is yes. If the answer is no, then ask, What can I do to spice it up without the sodium?

If you are worried about a dish being too bland, add an herb or spice you think will complement it (see Appendix A for our herb and spice guide). When a recipe calls for seasoned salts, use the plain spice instead of the salty version, for example, fresh minced garlic or garlic powder in place of garlic *salt*. Another strategy for reducing sodium but still getting flavor is to use small amounts of *moderately* salty seasonings such as chili powder, Parmesan cheese, and mustard instead of the high-sodium seasonings (see page 42) in your recipe. Use low-sodium sauces and marinades made primarily of herbs and spices, vinegar, honey, wine, or lemon juice instead of high-sodium bottled sauces, which are composed mainly of salt, MSG, and/or soy sauce. Meat tenderizers, steak sauces, and many bottled vegetable marinades are just colorful disguises for sodium. And remember, don't use salt substitutes, because they contain amounts of potassium that are dangerous for people with kidney disease. "Lite salt" is not low enough in sodium to make it healthy for you, so don't use it.

Unless you are experienced with baking, altering recipes for baked goods can be difficult. When evaluating whether a recipe fits your diet, keep in mind that self-rising flour contains added baking soda and salt and that flour contains some protein (6.5 g per ½ cup), while cornstarch has none.

Lessening the amount of potassium in a vegetable recipe means leaving out or reducing the amount of high-potassium vegetables, or substituting low-potassium vegetables for such high-potassium vegetables as tomatoes, potatoes, broccoli, and greens (see the table on page 53). Also, fresh tomatoes have less potassium than stewed tomatoes or tomato sauces and juices, so use fresh over canned when necessary. And remember, low-sodium canned tomatoes have less sodium, but they still have a lot of potassium, so moderate their use.

For a person on the protein-restricted diet, another way to alter recipes is to substitute vegetables for meats. For instance, slice a Portobello mushroom, which is large and "meaty," and substitute it for the meat in a recipe for a low-sodium marinated grilled beef sandwich. Or, in a recipe for a ground beef casserole, leave out the meat and add sautéed eggplant or bell peppers, squash, and onions.

An important part of meal planning and adapting recipes is figuring out how much of each of the recipe's ingredients you will be getting with each serving—for example, when you are preparing food for more than one person or making extra for freezing and saving. To calculate serving sizes, mentally divide the amount of each ingredient in the recipe by the number of servings the recipe makes. If you plan to eat more than one of the "official" servings, multiply the amount by the number of servings you will eat. For example, if a recipe calls for 1 cup of milk and makes six ½-cup servings, each serving contains ⅙ of a cup of milk. Since ½ of a cup contains about 4 grams of protein, you will get a little more than 1 gram from the milk part of the dish. Remember, though, if you eat 1 cup altogether you have consumed ⅓ of a cup of milk. Count it as 1 dairy serving or a little less.

Eating Out

In terms of diet and nutrition, eating out at restaurants, fast food or traditional sit-down, often poses diet problems. Sodium and protein seem to be everywhere! A single restaurant meal may contain thousands of milligrams of sodium and over 50 grams of protein. It is possible, though, to get a complete meal that contains a reasonable amount of sodium and protein from most restaurants.

First, take advantage of the fact that consumers today are more health-conscious than ever. Many restaurants have "healthy" menu items. These are a good place to begin when deciding what to order. In general, it is a good idea to avoid soups, heavily marinated items, and items with cream sauces, all of which contain too much sodium. Load up on salads, vegetables, and breads, but ask for dressings and butter on the side so you can monitor how much you add. (Bring packets of your own favorite low-sodium dressing just in case they don't offer appropriate selections.) A vegetable plate is an excellent way to minimize protein, but remember to ask for vegetables that have been or could be prepared without added salt or ham/bacon (which is salted pork).

Sometimes you may choose to eat meat when eating out. Before ordering, find out what the serving size of meat is, and clarify whether that is the cooked or raw weight. For example, in the phrase "an 8-ounce filet" the weight usually refers to the raw weight. Cooked, the meat will be more like 6 ounces (see formula on page 70). Most people on protein-restricted diets should not eat this much protein in one day, much less in one meal. For those on dialysis, this serving may be appropriate, but make sure to consider what else you have had that day to see how much more protein you can fit into your meal plan. If the amount of meat included in the dish will put you over your daily protein allowance, you can ask that part of the meat entrée be wrapped up beforehand and you can save it for the next day's meals. Smaller servings can also sometimes be requested.

How both meat and vegetable dishes are prepared is important as well. The breading on many baked and fried foods usually contains added salt, as do marinades. Grilled items will be quite tasty even when you ask for the marinade and/or sauces to be left off. Poached and broiled items, on the other hand, tend to be bland if salty sauces and marinades are not added, though low-sodium spices can certainly be added to enhance them. Don't hesitate to bring your own spice mix to a restaurant so you can spice up the food you order if it needs it.

Many people find themselves eating in fast-food restaurants a lot. In general, we recommend avoiding fast-food restaurants as much as possible. It is very difficult to get a truly healthy meal at one. When you do need to stop and have a meal or a snack, order just enough food to tide you over. Salads are a wise choice, but do not get the one with deli meat and cheese (often called a chef salad). Get one with just salad greens and vegetables or one with sliced grilled chicken, if appropriate to your diet. Order them with low-sodium and/or low-fat dressings when they are available.

Another reasonable fast-food choice is a plain meat entrée instead of an elaborate specialty item. For example, have a plain hamburger instead of a double decker with cheese, special sauce, and pickles. Have a plain beef taco or two instead of an elaborate marinated chicken enchilada platter. As a side dish, try a small order of un-salted french fries (it will take them a few minutes more), and share them if possible. Another option is low-fat frozen ice cream or ice milk (generally frozen yogurt contains high amounts of phosphorus). Have a small cone for a snack or as a dessert. On the other hand, avoid fried fruit pies; they are high in sodium.

Today, another option if you want food fast is to go to a large grocery store in your area. Pick up something healthy to snack on or, if you are lucky, put together the meal of your choice. Many stores are now stocking salad and hot bars where you can quickly assemble a meal that includes some healthy choices.

We encourage you to find healthy places to eat. The easiest place is at home, but no one can or wants to eat at home all of the time. Eating out, and even occasionally splurging, are choices you have. Just remember that where food is likely to be a center of attention, you need to be prepared to implement the guidelines of the renal nutrition plan you now know. If you splurge at one meal, proudly return to your diet ideals and do not get caught up in feelings of guilt or resentment about your diet. Make it yours!

Some things you can do to minimize the risk of getting stuck away from home, and hungry, with foods that do not fit your needs:

- Choose carefully where and what you eat. Find places that can accommodate special requests; call around to identify them.
- Look for items on restaurant menus marked "healthy"—but clarify with your server what it means.
- Ask that no salty seasonings be added to your food. Be explicit as to what that includes (for

example, Chinese food contains sodium added as MSG and soy sauce), and be prepared to wait a little longer for your items.

- Eat a small snack before going out so that you will not order too much food or stuff yourself.

- For cookouts, bring your own preweighed items for the grill. Mark your items with food coloring or toothpicks so they do not get mixed up with the others.

- If you are attending a special event at which a meal is provided, contact the event coordinator in advance and request that a special meal (for example, low sodium or vegetarian) be provided for you if at all possible.

- If you are going to someone else's house to eat, call them ahead of time and explain that you may not be able to eat some foods but that they should not be offended; it is because of your health condition. They will probably even offer to prepare some of the foods a little differently—for instance, with no added salt.

- For potlucks, make sure that you bring an item you can eat a lot of.

- Don't forget to call airlines to reserve special meals when you are flying. Or take your own meal and/or snack. (Don't eat those salted peanuts or pretzels they give out!)

- When you are traveling, pack healthy snacks such as fruit, low-sodium crackers and bread, and raw vegetable pieces. If you will be traveling around mealtime, pack sandwiches for you and your family. Bring a cooler to keep everything fresh.

Chapter Seven

Strategies for Change

Just about the most difficult part of this diet is that it requires most people to make significant changes in what they eat. Eating habits are ingrained in many ways, culturally and psychologically. And like changing anything that we are comfortable with, changing our diet is too often a negative experience. Many are not fully successful at implementing changes. We have come up with some strategies that will make the transition to this new, healthy way of eating easier and make it more likely that you will succeed. You will certainly be happy with the result if you do!

Number 1: Consider the Options

This is the principle that says, "By choosing this way, I am forgoing another, different way." If you are mindful of your choice—for example, unsalted crackers over salted potato chips—then the choice has given you power. If you are unaware of the other choices available to you, then you are powerless in your choices. Considering the options is about having the information to make conscious choices. In fact, you began that process when you picked up this book. You are heading in the right direction.

There is no way we can tell you *all* of your options. So how can you go about expanding your choices further? One of the best ways is to find out what foods are readily available to you. Set aside a few hours on one or several days and spend them perusing the overflowing shelves of the grocery store where you normally shop, reading and getting familiar with the information on the nutrition labels, the special claims, and the food ingredients. With all the new guidelines you have to consider—protein requirement or restriction, sodium and potassium restriction, and phosphorus management—you can really start to evaluate the value or realize the worthlessness of certain foods.

It is important to evaluate foods in many different ways. How will this food fit into my renal diet guidelines? How might I incorporate it into dishes and meals? How might it suit my palate? You are guaranteed to be both surprised and pleased at what you find on nutrition labels. Make knowing nutritional information a hobby of yours. That way you will know your options and choices, and that will give you power over your diet. It will also make eating according to our recommendations a fun challenge instead of an intimidating chore.

Number 2: Plan Ahead

Planning requires foresight. Plan ahead is the principle that says, "If I have prepared for what is ahead of me, my needs will likely be met when that time comes." By allowing you to influence what happens to you, planning frees you from reactions—such as picking up the salt shaker—

that oppose your dietary goals. For instance, if you plan *how* to make the green beans for dinner taste good using herbs and spices rather than salt, you will be able to enjoy your meal and not risk getting frustrated by their blandness.

Especially when you are just beginning on the renal diet, each day you should map out exactly *what* you will eat, *how* you will prepare it, and even *when* and *where* and with *whom* you will eat it. (And changing your plans is always your prerogative.) Once you get in the habit of planning meals it will become natural, and you will get to be so efficient that you will hardly notice the effort. The investment is small and the rewards are great. In the grand scheme, spending 15 minutes a day to plan meals is nothing. If you have a significant other, you must find a time when you can sit down together to plan meals—for example, while you eat breakfast or just before dinner.

Plan meals that you can look forward to. (Have your favorite meals most often. Variety is important, but there is no reason to limit your favorites as long as they are very healthy, too.) Sketch out several days at a time so you can make use of a grocery list then firm up your plans each day. By planning your meals ahead of time and shopping by a list, you begin to see what is important for you to buy and what you buy (and eat) simply out of habit.

In addition to facilitating your diet, the exercise of conscious meal planning can improve your concentration and mental agility, and even improve relationships with loved ones with whom you plan meals. And in general it allows you to avoid the stress and pitfalls of being hungry and having no meal planned.

Number 3: Assert Yourself

Asserting yourself is about making sure you can implement the plan you make. "If I do not let my needs be known, they may be ignored" is the principle here. Dr. Bernie S. Siegel, former cancer surgeon and author of the bestselling *Love, Medicine & Miracles,* reports finding that it is the patients who cause the most "trouble" that do the best. Asserting yourself is important anyplace you have needs—at home, on the job, in restaurants, at the doctor's office, in the hospital. If people cannot help you, they will let you know.

A great place to start practicing is in a restaurant. First, you should use the first two strategies discussed above to choose (or approve, if it was picked by someone else) the restaurant you will go to. Consider your options by getting recommendations from others and finding out yourself, firsthand, whether the restaurant can make some foods to order or serves dishes that meet your diet specifications. Plan ahead by eating light meals for breakfast and lunch, and, if appropriate, call the restaurant to remind them of your reservation and your special dietary needs. You have begun the process of asserting yourself by taking these actions.

Once in the restaurant, make a point of telling your server that you will need a few minutes of his or her time to ask some questions about the menu items. That way your server will come to your table ready to talk rather than rushed to get your order. You may have to wait a few minutes longer than other customers, but by asserting your needs you will get the full attention of your server.

When your order arrives, confirm with your server that it was prepared the way you specified. If your server is not absolutely sure, ask him or her to check with the kitchen. If, upon tasting the food, you feel that it was not prepared correctly, send it back. Though these things might be a hassle for your server, it is not your responsibility to suffer for the mistakes of the restaurant. Protect yourself by asserting your needs, and you will maintain your healthy way of eating even when eating out. Blindly accept what is given to you, and you may disrupt your health. If it makes you feel better about "imposing" on your server, leave him or her a generous tip. The majority of the time everything will turn out positively anyway.

Number 4: Remember Your Goal—Keeping Healthy

Remember-your-goal is about motivation. This principle says, "If I am motivated, my goals will come naturally." In terms of health, motivation comes from seeing your health improve.

The best way to track your improvements is to keep a private nutrition and health journal. You don't have to have a fancy notebook or write well enough for anybody but you to read. A simple notebook that you feel comfortable writing in will do best.

Jot down what you eat, everything or selectively. Keep track of how much protein you eat each day. Record your weight daily. (Weigh at approximately the same time each day.) Follow the patterns between water weight gain and high sodium consumption. It will inspire you to watch your sodium carefully. Record health symptoms, including itchy skin (phosphorus overload). Record the impact of dialysis sessions, exercise, meals out, or social interactions with others. Write down what you learn from your physician and dietitian. And, most importantly, record how you feel, physically and mentally. Your health journal can be a vehicle for getting yourself motivated. It is also a way for you to see what changes in diet and lifestyle have the most impact on your health. Remember, your goal is keeping healthy.

Chapter Eight

Other Health Matters

I n this chapter, we will briefly discuss other areas of health that relate to kidney disease. You now know that following a proper diet can slow progression of your disease. You should also know that exercising and maintaining a healthy body weight will help. Your ability to cope with your disease through health-care providers and social support also affect your overall health.

Exercise

Exercise can be beneficial in many ways. It improves appetite, reduces muscle wasting, increases muscle and bone strength, allows for better blood pressure and weight control, increases energy level, improves sleep and one's feeling of well-being, enhances the utilization of glucose (which is especially important for diabetics), and can lower blood cholesterol levels.

You don't have to get fancy. Examples are walking, swimming, lifting weights. Begin at a low intensity for your first workouts. Then challenge yourself to work a little harder each time. Plan how long you will go, and stop when it is time. If you felt good, plan to go longer the next time. Work toward 30-minute workouts. Every other day (3 to 4 times a week) is an excellent goal.

The first step to implementing an exercise plan is to approve it with your physician. He or she may want you to take some tests to determine at what level you should start. Keep in mind that exercise can potentially aggravate your condition if you have not also changed your diet or if you are not taking prescribed medications.

Don't wait another minute before making a plan of action. You will feel healthier almost immediately. Be sure to record your progress in your health journal. It will motivate you to keep up your exercise plan and to keep up the good work on controlling your diet.

Body Weight

In addition to protein restriction, maintaining a healthy weight is a very important part of preventing the advancement of kidney disease. Carrying extra weight around puts added stress on your kidneys and has been shown to be related to an increased risk of premature death in the general population. Thus, for people with renal insufficiency who are diagnosed early, weight loss, when necessary, can be of benefit.

The first set of weights given in the table on page 85 corresponds to a maximum body weight that can be considered healthy. If you are overweight, use this value as a goal (lose incrementally if you are more than 20 percent over this weight). For those who reach a healthy weight, the value in the second set of weights corresponds to an even healthier weight that you can use as a goal in further weight loss.

Healthy Weight Chart

Height	Healthy Weight Maximum (lbs)	Healthier Weight Maximum (lbs)
4'10"	119	109
4'11"	124	114
5'0"	128	118
5'1"	132	121
5'2"	136	125
5'3"	141	130
5'4"	145	133
5'5"	150	138
5'6"	155	143
5'7"	159	146
5'8"	164	151
5'9"	169	155
5'10"	174	160
5'11"	179	165
6'0"	184	169
6'1"	189	174
6'2"	194	178
6'3"	200	184

From the American Health Foundation's Expert Panel on Healthy Weight

As opposed to people who have early disease and are not on dialysis, for people with advanced kidney failure, particularly those on dialysis, healthy weight loss is very difficult because of altered metabolism and kidney function. Protein wasting is common during weight loss in this group. "Dieting" in the sense of trying to lose a significant amount of weight can be dangerous if not monitored by a dietitian or physician.

Make sure you recognize the difference between intentional weight loss (accomplished through conscious changes in your eating and exercise patterns) and unintentional weight loss (suffered because of losses in appetite). Unintentional weight loss is likely to be accompanied by overall malnutrition. Consciously monitor your weight to make sure it does not go down when you don't expect it to.

Talking with Health-Care Professionals

Health care has many facets. Medical diagnosis, treatment, nutritional and mental health counseling, and help with medications are just a few of the areas in which a proper health-care system works. It is likely that you will need the services of many different health-care professionals at various times during the course of your disease.

In addition to a physician or medical doctor (M.D.), other important health-care professionals may include a physician assistant (P.A.); registered nurse (R.N.) and licensed practical nurse (L.P.N.); registered dietitian (R.D.) and licensed dietitian nutritionist (L.D.N.); pharmacists and social workers. In most cases, if one of the health-care professionals you see cannot help you directly, he or she can refer you to another.

The same principles that apply to making changes in your diet (see Chapter Seven) apply to dealing with the health-care system through which you are being treated. First, know your options. Find out from your physician or the staff at the clinic you go to what resources are available. Is there a registered dietitian you could see? Or a social worker you could see for a problem with financial matters? Most times your physician has to make recommendations for you to see them. Plan ahead and assert yourself when presenting your needs.

Plan to talk to your physician or physician assistant during your next visit about the issues that are important to you. Make a list so you won't forget. Don't just imply that you want to talk to a mental-health professional; say it outright.

Remember your goal—keeping healthy. Inform your health-care professionals of any changes in your condition. With regard to nutrition, this includes changes in taste, appetite, and body weight.

Work, Volunteerism, and Social Support

There are many life-enhancing activities a person with kidney disease can engage in. Illnesses tend to isolate people, and that is just the opposite of what they need. Continuing work after diagnosis is associated with better long-term health. When work is out of the question—perhaps the work you have done all your life is too strenuous for you now—think about volunteering. You can spend time tutoring or playing with children. Volunteer at a soup kitchen or for a political campaign. The pressure will be significantly less than at a job, and the sense of fulfillment as good or better. Engaging in activities that make you feel useful motivates you to keep healthy.

Support groups are another activity that fosters social support. A group for people with kidney disease would be ideal, but being in a group with people who are struggling with practically any illness will be of benefit. Support groups help for many reasons, the most important of which is learning that you are not alone. You can find out about local support groups through your local dialysis center or through some of the national resources listed in the back of this book.

The most important support group for many is the family. If there are bad feelings or misunderstandings among your family members, seek counseling for yourself or your family so that the problems can be resolved and the focus put back on each other's well-being.

Chapter Nine

Recipes

The chefs at Innovations, the Stedman Center's restaurant, have been making healthy food for people with chronic diseases for many years. The recipes included in this chapter are kidney-smart. They are easily incorporated into your meal-planning guidelines and contain minimum amounts of sodium. Potassium is also limited but varies a great deal from recipe to recipe, so pay attention to how the potassium in each recipe fits into your meal plan. A little over half the main dishes are meat or fish based. For those on protein restriction, remember that an easy way to limit protein is to eat meat, fish, or eggs at only one meal each day.

If you do not enjoy cooking all the time, double recipes and freeze the extra servings for later on. You are at the helm in your kitchen. Follow these recipes closely the first time, then make healthy adjustments for your own taste the next.

Pesto Breadsticks

2	hot dog buns
1	tablespoon sesame seeds
1	teaspoon dried basil
1	teaspoon dried parsley
1	teaspoon garlic powder
1	tablespoon grated Parmesan cheese
4	tablespoons olive oil

Preheat the oven to 350°F. Split each bun, then cut each half in three lengthwise. In a shallow pan, combine the sesame seeds, basil, parsley, garlic powder, and Parmesan. Lightly brush a piece of bread with oil, roll it in the sesame mixture, and place it on a baking sheet. Repeat with the other pieces. Bake about 15 minutes, or until crisp.

Variations: For Poppy Breadsticks, roll the bread in 2 tablespoons poppy seeds; for Spicy Breadsticks, roll it in a mixture of ½ teaspoon chili powder, ¼ teaspoon garlic powder, and a pinch of cayenne; for Dessert Breadsticks, sprinkle with a mixture of 2 tablespoons brown sugar, ½ teaspoon cinnamon, and ⅛ teaspoon nutmeg.

Yield: 6 2-piece servings

Calories per serving: 121
Protein: 2 g
Sodium: 95 mg
Potassium: 45 mg
Phosphorus: 34 mg

Snack Mix

- ½   cup Corn Chex
- ½   cup Rice Chex
- 1   cup unsalted air-popped popcorn
- 1   cup unsalted pretzel sticks
- ¼   cup unsalted butter, melted
- ¼   teaspoon garlic powder
- ¼   teaspoon onion powder
- ⅛   teaspoon chili powder, or to taste
- 1   tablespoon grated Parmesan cheese

Combine the corn and rice cereal, popcorn, and pretzels in a large bowl. Add the garlic powder, onion powder, and chili powder to the melted butter. Slowly pour the spiced butter over the cereal-and-popcorn mixture while stirring with a large wooden spoon. Sprinkle on the Parmesan and toss.

Yield: 6 servings

Calories per serving: 132
Protein: 1.8 g
Sodium: 69.6 mg
Potassium: 29 mg
Phosphorus: 28 mg

Fruit Salad with Poppyseed Dressing

4	cups torn lettuce leaves
1	cup red seedless grapes
1	cup grapefruit sections
1	cup orange sections
1	cup sliced strawberries
¼	cup fruit juice
1	tablespoon rice-wine or other mild vinegar
1	tablespoon canola or other vegetable oil
2	teaspoons honey
2	teaspoons poppy seeds
1	teaspoon mustard

Divide the lettuce, grapes, orange sections, and strawberries among four plates. To make the dressing, combine the fruit juice, vinegar, oil, honey, poppy seeds, and mustard in a small bowl and whisk to blend. Dress the salad and serve chilled.

Variation: For a salad somewhat lower in potassium, substitute sliced pears for the grapefruit and tangerine sections for the orange. This low-protein salad can be turned into a high-protein meal by adding pieces of chicken or pork.

Yield: 4 servings

Calories per serving: 144
Protein: 2.3 g
Sodium: 23 mg
Potassium: 434 mg
Phosphorus: 51 mg

Dill Tuna-Noodle Chowder

4	tablespoons unsalted margarine or butter
¼	cup flour
2	cups low-sodium fish stock or chicken broth
2	cups low-fat milk
2	cups uncooked egg noodles
1	medium onion, chopped
1	medium carrot, chopped
	6½-ounce can low-sodium, water-packed tuna, drained
1	tablespoon lemon juice or white vinegar
2	tablespoons fresh dill or 1 teaspoon dried

Melt the margarine in a large saucepan set over medium heat. Stir in the flour and cook 3 minutes, stirring. Gradually stir in the stock and milk. When the mixture starts to thicken, add the noodles, onion, and carrot. Turn down the heat, cover, and simmer 15 minutes, or until the noodles and vegetables soften. Add the tuna and cook about 5 minutes, or until heated through. Remove from the heat, stir in the lemon juice and dill, and serve.

Yield: 8 1-cup servings

Calories per serving: 182
Protein: 10 g
Sodium: 48 mg
Potassium: 227 mg
Phosphorus: 157 mg

Low-Sodium Mayonnaise

1   egg yolk
2   tablespoons lemon juice
¼   teaspoon mustard
1   cup canola oil
¼   teaspoon paprika

Put the egg yolk, lemon juice, and mustard in the bowl of a blender and process to combine. Add the oil and blend at medium speed about 1 minute, or until creamy. Mix in the paprika. Store in a covered container in the refrigerator.

Yield: 20 1-tablespoon servings

Calories per serving: 100
Protein: 0.2 g
Sodium: 1 mg
Potassium: 3 mg
Phosphorus: 4 mg

Vinaigrette

1	cup water
1	tablespoon cornstarch
1	teaspoon mustard
1	clove garlic, minced
½	cup red-wine vinegar
2	teaspoons ground black pepper
¼	cup olive oil

Bring the water to a boil in a small saucepan. Remove from the heat and add the cornstarch, stirring until it is dissolved. Return the pan to low heat and simmer until the mixture thickens, stirring to prevent lumps. Remove from the heat and set aside. In a small bowl, combine the mustard, garlic, vinegar, pepper, and oil. Stir this into the cornstarch mixture. Store in a covered container in the refrigerator.

Yield: 16 2-tablespoon servings

Calories per serving: 34
Protein: 0 g
Sodium: 4 mg
Potassium: 12 mg
Phosphorus: 2 mg

Cool Cucumber Salad

¾   cup low-fat sour cream
2   teaspoons rice-wine or other mild vinegar
½   clove garlic, minced, or ¼ teaspoon garlic
     powder
1   tablespoon chopped fresh mint
2   medium cucumbers, peeled and diced
3   lettuce leaves

Combine the sour cream, vinegar, garlic, and mint in a medium bowl. Stir in the cucumber. Cover with plastic wrap and refrigerate at least 3 hours. Serve on a lettuce leaf as a side salad.

Yield: 3 servings

Calories per serving: 98
Protein: 2.5 g
Sodium: 26 mg
Potassium: 228 mg
Phosphorus: 78 mg

Not-Just-For-Barbecue Sauce

6-ounce can low-sodium tomato paste
2 cloves garlic, minced
¾ cup water
¾ cup cider vinegar
2 tablespoons canola or other vegetable oil
2 tablespoons honey
4 teaspoons chili powder
½ teaspoon ground cumin
Dash Tabasco, or to taste

In a medium-sized stainless-steel saucepan, combine the tomato paste, garlic, and water. Bring to a boil, then lower the heat and simmer, uncovered, 2 to 3 minutes, stirring continually. Add the vinegar, oil, honey, chili powder, and cumin, and simmer 15 minutes more, stirring occasionally. Add the Tabasco. Store in a covered container in the refrigerator.

In addition to barbecuing, use as a dipping sauce or as a sauce for rice or potatoes.

Yield: 12 3-tablespoon servings

Calories per serving: 49
Protein: 0.7 g
Sodium: 18 mg
Potassium: 168 mg
Phosphorus: 16 mg

Stuffed French Toast

¼ cup low-fat cottage cheese
½ cup unsweetened applesauce
⅛ teaspoon ground clove or nutmeg
1 egg
1 tablespoon water or low-fat milk
¼ teaspoon cinnamon
2 teaspoons unsalted margarine or butter
2 pieces day-old or lightly toasted low-sodium bread
1 teaspoon powdered sugar

Combine the cottage cheese, applesauce, and clove in a microwave-safe container and set aside. In a shallow bowl, beat the egg, water, and cinnamon until well-mixed. Heat the margarine in a skillet set over medium heat. Dip the bread in the egg mixture, coating both sides, and place it in the skillet. When it is brown on one side, flip it and brown the other. Meanwhile, microwave the cottage cheese mixture at full power 1 to 2 minutes, or until warm through. Spread the filling on one piece of the bread and top it with the other. Sprinkle with the powdered sugar and serve immediately.

Yield: 1 serving

Calories per serving: 336
Protein: 12 g
Sodium: 113 mg
Potassium: 239 mg
Phosphorus: 184 mg

Cinnamon-Apple Muffins

1¼	cups flour
1 ½	cups plus 2 tablespoons rolled oats
1	teaspoon cinnamon
1	teaspoon baking powder
¾	teaspoon baking soda
1	cup unsweetened applesauce
½	cup low-fat milk
½	cup packed brown sugar
1	egg white
3	tablespoons canola or other vegetable oil
½	medium apple, peeled and diced

Preheat the oven to 400°F. and line 12 medium muffin cups. In a medium bowl, combine the flour, 1½ cups of the oats, the cinnamon, baking powder, and baking soda. Add the applesauce, milk, sugar, egg white, and oil, and mix just to blend. Stir in the apple pieces. Fill the prepared muffin cups ¾ with batter. Sprinkle ½ teaspoon oats on top of each muffin. Bake 20 to 25 minutes, or until done. Serve warm. (Leftover muffins can be frozen and reheated in the microwave.)

Yield: 12 servings

Calories per serving: 160
Protein: 3.8 g
Sodium: 96 mg
Potassium: 115 mg
Phosphorus: 118 mg

Cinnamon Toast

- 1 tablespoon packed brown sugar
- ⅛ teaspoon cinnamon
- 1 tablespoon unsalted margarine or butter, melted
- 2 slices bread

Stir the sugar and cinnamon into the melted margarine to form a rich brown paste. Toast the bread and spread the mixture over the toast. Serve immediately.

Yield: 2 servings

Calories per serving: 144
Protein: 2.5 g
Sodium: 145 mg
Potassium: 48 mg
Phosphorus: 30 mg

Turkey-and-Vegetable Frittata

10	eggs
2	teaspoons chopped fresh basil
½	teaspoon dried oregano
2	tablespoons chopped fresh parsley
	Vegetable cooking spray
2	tablespoons olive or other vegetable oil
1	clove garlic, minced
¼	cup chopped scallion
1¼	pounds raw turkey breast, partially frozen for ease of cutting
1	small zucchini, diced
½	red bell pepper, diced
1	cup corn kernels, fresh or frozen
½	cup grated low-sodium cheddar cheese or ¼ cup regular
⅛	teaspoon ground black pepper

Preheat oven to 325°F. In a medium bowl, combine the eggs, basil, oregano, and parsley. Coat a large ovenproof casserole with spray oil and pour the egg mixture into it. Cut the turkey into ½-inch dice. In a large skillet, heat 1 tablespoon of the oil over low heat. Add the garlic, scallion, and turkey and sauté, stirring continually, about 10 minutes, or until the turkey is cooked through. Add the turkey mixture to the egg in the casserole. Using the same skillet, heat the remaining 1 tablespoon oil and add the zucchini, bell pepper, and corn. Cover and cook over medium heat about 7 minutes, stirring occasionally, until the vegetables soften. Add the vegetable mixture to the casserole. Stir the ingredients in the casserole and bake about 30 minutes, or until the eggs are set (they can still be moist on top). Sprinkle the cheese and pepper on top and cook 5 minutes more or until cheese is melted. Serve immediately.

Yield: 6 servings

Calories per serving: 267
Protein: 22 g
Sodium: 125 mg
Potassium: 294 mg
Phosphorus: 272 mg

Flounder Stuffed with Mushrooms

2 teaspoons olive or other vegetable oil
⅓ pound fresh mushrooms, sliced (about 2 cups)
4 shiitake mushrooms, stems removed, sliced
½ cup chopped scallion
½ teaspoon fresh minced ginger or ¼ teaspoon dried
2 tablespoons chopped fresh parsley or 1 tablespoon dried
4 flounder fillets, about 4 ounces each
1 tablespoon lemon juice
Ground black pepper
⅓ cup white wine or water

Preheat the oven to 350°F. Heat the oil in a medium skillet set over medium heat. Add the mushrooms, shiitakes, scallion, and ginger and sauté until the mushrooms shrink and darken. Remove from the heat and stir in the parsley. Sprinkle the fish with lemon juice and pepper. Place a mound of stuffing at one end of each fillet and roll them up. Place the rolls seam-side down in a shallow baking dish and add the wine. Bake 25 minutes, or until the fish is cooked through. Serve immediately.

Yield: 4 servings

Calories per serving: 162
Protein: 23 g
Sodium: 98 mg
Potassium: 636 mg
Phosphorus: 262 mg

Fish Cakes

1¼	pounds fillet of salmon or other fish
1	egg white
1	medium onion, minced
¼	cup chopped green bell pepper
¼	cup chopped scallion
2	teaspoons mustard
2	tablespoons plain low-fat yogurt, preferably drained for 2 hours in paper towel
	Flour for dusting
3	teaspoons peanut or other vegetable oil

In a food processor, briefly process 1 pound of the fish. Dice the remaining ¼ pound by hand. In a large bowl, mix together all the fish and the egg white. Stir in the onion, bell pepper, scallion, mustard, and yogurt. Dust an ungreased baking sheet with flour. Form the fish mixture into 6 cakes and place them on the baking sheet. Dust the tops with flour. In a medium skillet, heat 1 teaspoon of the oil over medium heat. Lightly brown both sides of the cakes two at a time. Use 1 teaspoon oil for each of the other two pairs. If the fish cakes have not cooked through completely, cover the skillet and cook over medium-low heat until they are done.

Yield: 6 servings

Calories per serving: 155
Protein: 20 g
Sodium: 99 mg
Potassium: 378 mg
Phosphorus: 238 mg

Spicy Coated Chicken Breast

½ cup rolled oats
½ teaspoon chili powder
¼ teaspoon ground black pepper
1 teaspoon paprika
1 tablespoon chopped fresh parsley or 1 teaspoon dried
2 eggs
1 tablespoon water
2 whole skinless boneless chicken breasts, split
4 teaspoons unsalted margarine, melted

Preheat oven to 425°F. Put the oats, chili powder, pepper, paprika, and parsley in a food processor and pulse until fine. Place the mixture in a shallow bowl. In another shallow bowl, beat the eggs with the water. Dip the chicken breasts first in the egg mixture, then in the oat mixture, and place them in a shallow baking pan. Drizzle the margarine on top and bake about 35 minutes, or until cooked through.

Yield: 4 servings

Calories per serving: 242
Protein: 32 g
Sodium: 113 mg
Potassium: 393 mg
Phosphorus: 328 mg

Pot Roast

	3-pound bottom round roast or brisket
2	garlic cloves, sliced
1	medium onion, sliced thin
1	cup red-wine vinegar
4	tablespoons unsalted margarine
2	cups strong brewed coffee (regular or decaffeinated)
2	cups water
1	pound carrots, peeled and cut into 1-inch pieces
12	pearl onions, peeled
¼	teaspoon ground black pepper, or to taste
2	tablespoons flour
¼	cup water

Trim all visible fat from the roast and place it in a large bowl. Make slits in the meat and insert the garlic slices in them. Arrange the sliced onion on top of the roast. Pour the vinegar over the meat, cover with plastic wrap, and allow to marinate 24 hours in the refrigerator, turning the roast several times. Drain the roast and pat dry with paper towels. Heat the margarine until almost boiling and pour it over the meat to brown it. Place the drained roast in a covered casserole or dutch oven. Add the coffee and water, bring to a boil, cover, and simmer 2 hours. Add the carrots, pearl onions, and pepper, and simmer 1 more hour, or until tender. Remove the roast from the pan. To make gravy, mix the flour with the water and add it to the cooking liquid. Cook over medium heat, stirring continually until thickened.

Yield: 12 4-ounce servings

Calories per serving: 243
Protein: 32 g
Sodium: 100 mg
Potassium: 464 mg
Phosphorus: 291 mg

East Indian Sautéed Chicken

4	tablespoons flour
¼	teaspoon ground cumin
¼	teaspoon ground coriander
¼	teaspoon ground black pepper
2	whole skinless boneless chicken breasts, split and cut into 1-inch strips
3	tablespoons olive or other vegetable oil

Combine the flour, cumin, coriander, and pepper in a shallow bowl. Put the chicken strips in the bowl and turn to coat with the flour mixture. In a large skillet, heat the oil over medium-high heat. Sauté the chicken, turning to brown all over. Reduce the heat and cover to finish cooking. Serve immediately with Saffron Rice (page 130). Keep in mind that the Saffron Rice recipe makes 6 servings.

Yield: 4 servings

Calories per serving: 248
Protein: 28 g
Sodium: 77 mg
Potassium: 314 mg
Phosphorus: 241 mg

Honey-Mustard Pork Tenderloin

¼ cup honey
2 tablespoons cider vinegar
2 tablespoons packed brown sugar
1 tablespoon mustard
½ teaspoon paprika
2 tablespoons unsalted margarine, melted
   (optional)
   1¼-pound pork tenderloin

Preheat the oven to 375°F. In a small bowl, combine the honey, vinegar, sugar, mustard, paprika, and margarine. Trim all visible fat from the meat, place it in a roasting pan just big enough to hold it, and pour the sauce over it. Roast 20 to 30 minutes, basting every 10 minutes, or until the temperature registers 160°F. on an instant-read thermometer. Slice thin and serve warm.

Yield: 6 3-ounce servings

Calories per serving: 215
Protein: 21 g
Sodium: 77 mg
Potassium: 363 mg
Phosphorus: 201 mg

Turkey Pot Pie

4	tablespoons unsalted margarine
3	tablespoons flour
	16-ounce can low-sodium chicken broth
1½	cups mixed frozen vegetables, such as peas, corn, and onion
1¼	pounds cooked white-meat turkey, diced
½	teaspoon dried thyme
⅛	teaspoon ground black pepper
1	teaspoon dried parsley
	Vegetable cooking spray
1	frozen pie crust, thawed
1	egg, lightly beaten
2	tablespoons water

Preheat the oven to 400°F. Melt the margarine in a medium saucepan set over medium heat. Add the flour and cook about 3 minutes, stirring continually. Gradually add the broth, stirring to remove any lumps. Increase the heat and bring to a light boil. Add the vegetables, reduce the heat, and simmer 10 minutes, stirring occasionally. Remove the pan from the heat and stir in the turkey, thyme, pepper, and parsley. Pour the mixture into a 4-inch deep, 1-quart casserole dish coated with spray oil. Remove the crust from its pan and cover the casserole with it. Poke holes in the top with a fork or knife to vent. Combine the egg and water in a small bowl, and brush the crust with it. Bake 45 minutes, or until the filling is bubbly and the top is browned. Allow to cool slightly before serving.

Yield: 7 servings

Calories per serving: 306
Protein: 22 g
Sodium: 236 mg
Potassium: 250 mg
Phosphorus: 178 mg

Chicken and Barley Salad

¼	cup pearl barley
1	medium stalk celery, diced
½	medium onion, diced
½	medium apple, peeled and diced
2	tablespoons plain low-fat yogurt
2	tablespoons low-fat milk
1	tablespoon chopped fresh parsley
1	tablespoon chopped fresh basil
1	tablespoon low-fat mayonnaise
1	clove garlic, minced
1	tablespoon lemon juice
2	teaspoons grated lemon zest
⅛	teaspoon ground black pepper
¾	pound cooked chicken breast, diced

Prepare the barley according to package instructions, omitting any added salt. In a large bowl, combine the celery, onion, apple, yogurt, milk, parsley, basil, mayonnaise, garlic, lemon juice, zest, and pepper. Add the chicken and toss to coat. Add well-drained barley to the chicken mixture and toss again. Serve at room temperature or chilled.

Yield: 4 servings

Calories per serving: 172
Protein: 22 g
Sodium: 100 mg
Potassium: 404 mg
Phosphorus: 228 mg

Vegetable Calzone

For the crust:

1	teaspoon sugar
¾	cup very warm water (between 105° and 115°F.)
1	package rapid-rise yeast
2¼	cups flour plus more as necessary

For the filling:

3	teaspoons canola or other vegetable oil
1	medium green bell pepper, diced
1	medium red or yellow bell pepper, diced
½	medium onion, diced
1	large zucchini, sliced thin
1½	cups broccoli florets
1	medium tomato, seeded and diced
½	teaspoon dried oregano
½	teaspoon dried basil
1	tablespoon dried parsley
4	teaspoons grated Parmesan cheese
	Vegetable cooking spray

Preheat the oven to 375°F. In a medium bowl, combine the sugar and water. Add the yeast and stir to dissolve. Let rest 5 minutes; the yeast should bubble. Place the 2¼ cups flour in a large bowl. Make a well in the center and slowly add the yeast mixture, mixing gently to form a dough. Knead the dough by hand 6 to 8 minutes, or until it is smooth and elastic. If the dough is too sticky, knead in a bit more flour. Lightly dust the ball of dough with flour, place it in a bowl, and cover with a towel or plastic wrap. Keep in a warm, draft-free place about 30 minutes, or until doubled in bulk. In a medium skillet, heat 1 teaspoon of the oil over medium heat. Add the green pepper, red pepper, and onion, and sauté until the onion is transluscent. Add the zucchini, broccoli, tomato, oregano, basil, and parsley. Cover and cook about 5 minutes, or until the vegetables start to soften. Punch down the dough and divide it into 4 balls. (Keep each ball covered with plastic wrap until you are ready to roll it out.) Prepare each crust by placing a ball of dough on a lightly floured surface, rolling it out into an 8-inch circle with a lightly floured rolling pin, and pricking it all over with a fork. Brush the dough with ½ teaspoon of the remaining 2 teaspoons oil and sprinkle with 1 teaspoon of the Parmesan. Place one quarter of the vegetable mixture on half the circle and fold to form a half-moon shape. Press the edges together to seal and poke a few holes in the top with a fork. Place on a baking sheet coated with spray oil. Repeat with the rest of the dough and vegetables. Bake 25 to 30 minutes, or until golden brown.

Yield: 4 servings

Calories per serving: 341
Protein: 11 g
Sodium: 56 mg
Potassium: 457 mg
Phosphorus: 166 mg

Stewed Vegetables

2   large baking potatoes, peeled and cut into
    1-inch cubes
½   pound carrots, peeled and sliced
½   pound green beans, cut into 2-inch pieces
2   tablespoons canola or other vegetable oil
2   small onions, peeled and quartered
1   medium green bell pepper, diced
2   chili peppers, seeded and chopped
2   teaspoons grated fresh ginger or 1 teaspoon
    dried
2   cloves garlic, minced
½   teaspoon ground black pepper
7   scallions, chopped

Soak the potatoes in water overnight to remove some of
the potassium. Bring a large saucepan of water to a boil
and add the potatoes, carrots, and green beans. Cook 7
minutes, drain, and set aside. In the same saucepan, heat
the oil over medium-high heat. Add the onion, green
pepper, and chili pepper. Sauté 5 minutes, stirring constantly. Add the ginger, garlic, black pepper, and scallion.
Stir well, then add the reserved vegetables and stir again.
Cover and cook over low heat, stirring occasionally, 8 to
10 minutes, or until the vegetables are tender.

Yield: 4 servings

Calories per serving: 215
Protein: 5 g
Sodium: 34 mg
Potassium: 846 mg (unleached potatoes)
Phosphorus: 123 mg

Summertime Vegetable and Orzo Salad

¼	cup red-wine vinegar
⅓	cup canola or other vegetable oil
2	tablespoons lemon juice
1	clove garlic, minced
¼	cup chopped fresh basil
2	tablespoons chopped fresh parsley
1	medium zucchini, sliced thin
2	medium tomatoes, seeded and diced
2	small or 1 large cucumber, peeled and diced
½	medium onion, diced
¼	cup grated Parmesan cheese
2	cups cooked orzo or other small pasta, prepared without added salt

Put the vinegar, oil, lemon juice, garlic, basil, and parsley in a jar with a tight-fitting lid and shake well. Put the zucchini, tomato, cucumber, onion, and Parmesan in a large bowl, add the dressing and the orzo, and toss lightly. Cover with plastic wrap and refrigerate at least 2 hours, or overnight. Serve chilled or at room temperature.

Yield: 4 servings

Calories per serving: 159
Protein: 6 g
Sodium: 101 mg
Potassium: 308 mg
Phosphorus: 107 mg

Eggplant Manicotti

- 1 medium eggplant
- 2 tablespoons canola or other vegetable oil
- 2 cloves garlic, minced
- 2 tablespoons chopped scallion
- 1 medium zucchini, diced
- ½ teaspoon dried oregano
- 1 tablespoon chopped fresh parsley
- ½ teaspoon dried thyme
- ¼ teaspoon ground black pepper
- 6 manicotti shells, cooked al dente without added salt
  Vegetable cooking spray
- 4 slices tomato

Preheat the oven to 350°F. Cut the eggplant in half lengthwise and place the halves cut part down on a cookie sheet. Pierce the skin several times with a fork. Bake 30 to 45 minutes, or until a fork inserts easily into the flesh. While the eggplant is baking, heat the oil in a skillet set over medium-low heat. Add the garlic and cook 1 minute, stirring continually. Add the scallion, zucchini, oregano, parsley, thyme, and pepper. Increase the heat to medium and cook 5 to 7 minutes, or until the zucchini is done. When the eggplant is cool enough to handle, scoop out the flesh and add it to the vegetables in the skillet. Spoon the mixture into the manicotti shells and arrange them in a shallow baking dish coated with spray oil. Top with the tomato slices and bake 10 minutes, or until heated through.

Yield: 3 servings

Calories per serving: 199
Protein: 5 g
Sodium: 12 mg
Potassium: 501 mg
Phosphorus: 96 mg

Creamy Mushroom-and-Rice Casserole

3	tablespoons unsalted butter or margarine
½	pound mushrooms, sliced
¼	cup chopped scallion
¼	cup flour
2	tablespoons fresh chopped parsley or 1 tablespoon dried
1	tablespoon fresh chopped basil or ½ tablespoon dried
1	tablespoon mustard
⅛	teaspoon ground black pepper
1	cup rice
1	cup nondairy creamer
1	cup water

Heat the butter in a large skillet set over medium heat. Add the mushrooms and scallion, and cook about 4 minutes, or until the mushrooms darken and shrink a bit. Add the flour, parsley, basil, mustard, and pepper, and stir well. Add the rice, creamer, and water. Bring to a boil, cover, and reduce the heat. Simmer 20 minutes, or until all the liquid has been absorbed. Serve warm.

Yield: 6 servings

Calories per serving: 247
Protein: 4 g
Sodium: 57 mg
Potassium: 260 mg
Phosphorus: 108 mg

Creole Stew

Low-protein version:
> Omit meat or seafood

High-protein version:
- ¾   pound diced chicken, turkey, pork, or fish, or whole scallops or peeled shrimp

- 2   tablespoons canola or other vegetable oil
- 2   cloves garlic, minced
- 1   large red onion, chopped
- 1   stalk celery, sliced ¼-inch thick on the diagonal
- ½   cup rice
- 1   large green bell pepper, chopped
- 5   small pods okra, sliced
- 1   medium yellow squash, chopped
     20-ounce can low-sodium tomatoes
- 2   teaspoons paprika
- 1   tablespoon Worcestershire sauce
     Dash Tabasco, or to taste

Heat the oil in a large skillet set over medium heat. Add the garlic, onion, and celery, and sauté 4 minutes. Add the rice, green pepper, okra, squash, tomatoes, paprika, Worcestershire, and Tabasco. Add the meat or seafood, if using. Cover and slowly simmer 3 hours, stirring occasionally. Serve hot.

Yield: 6 servings

Low-protein version
Calories per serving: 150
Protein: 3 g
Sodium: 52 mg
Potassium: 453 mg
Phosphorus: 69 mg

High-protein version (using shrimp)
Calories per serving: 206
Protein: 15 g
Sodium: 179 mg
Potassium: 556 mg
Phosphorus: 147 mg

Tempura with Sweet-and-Sour Sauce

Low-protein version:

    6   cups cut-up raw vegetables, such as zucchini, mushrooms, cauliflower, onion, broccoli, green or red bell pepper, asparagus, and carrot

High-protein version:

    2½   pounds thin-sliced meat, such as chicken, pork loin, and beef tips, or fish or firm tofu, or whole shelled shrimp, clams, or oysters, plus ½ cup chopped vegetables, such as green pepper, onion, and carrot, plus ¼ cup pineapple chunks for the sauce

For the tempura:

        Juice of 1 lemon
    1   egg
    1   cup water
    1   cup flour
    ½   teaspoon ground ginger
        Vegetable oil for deep-frying

For the sauce:

    ½   cup pineapple juice or liquid from canned pineapple
    1   tablespoon cornstarch
    ¼   cup cider vinegar
    ½   cup packed brown sugar
    1   tablespoon toasted sesame oil

For the batter, put the lemon juice in a large bowl and beat in the egg and water. Add the flour a bit at a time, stirring until smooth after each addition. The batter should be thin but should coat the spoon; add a bit more flour or water as necessary. Stir in the ginger. Refrigerate at least 15 minutes. For the sauce, combine the pineapple juice and cornstarch in a small saucepan. Heat gently until the cornstarch dissolves and the mixture thickens a bit. Add the vinegar, sugar, and sesame oil, and stir well. For vegetable tempura, remove the sauce from the heat now. For meat, seafood, or tofu tempura, add the ½ cup chopped vegetables, cover, and simmer 15 minutes, or until the carrots are tender. Stir in the pineapple. In a deep skillet, heat 1½ to 2 inches of oil to 325°F., or until a drop of water quickly sizzles away. One at a time, dip vegetable or meat, seafood, or tofu pieces into the chilled batter and drop them carefully into the hot oil. Cook several pieces at once but do not crowd the pan. Turn the pieces at least once during the cooking. Cook until crisp and brown on the outside. Remove the pieces, place on paper towels to drain, and keep warm. Serve immediately. For vegetable tempura, use the sauce for dipping; for meat, seafood, or tofu tempura, cover with the warm sauce.

Yield: 6 servings

Low-protein version
Calories per serving: 338
Protein: 6 g
Sodium: 39 mg
Potassium: 511 mg
Phosphorus: 128 mg

High-protein version (using half chicken and half shrimp)
Calories per serving: 420
Protein: 29 g

Sodium: 143 mg
Potassium: 307 mg
Phosphorus: 281 mg

Sauce with added vegetables
Calories per serving: 92.3
Protein: 0 g
Sodium: 10 mg
Potassium: 112 mg
Phosphorus: 10 mg

Peas-and-Potato Mash

Low-protein version:

3	medium all-purpose potatoes, peeled and cubed
1	cup cooked peas, fresh or frozen

High-protein version:

1	medium all-purpose potato, peeled and cubed
¾	cup cooked peas, fresh or frozen
1	pound lean ground beef
1	tablespoon unsalted margarine
2	tablespoons chopped fresh cilantro
3	tablespoons chopped scallion
	Pinch cayenne, or to taste
½	teaspoon sugar
¼	teaspoon ground turmeric

Soak the potatoes in water overnight to remove some of the potassium. Put the potatoes in a large saucepan, add water to cover, and boil 15 to 20 minutes, or until tender. Drain and return the potatoes to the saucepan. Add the peas, margarine, cilantro, scallion, cayenne, and sugar, and mash to the desired consistency. For the low-protein version, add the turmeric and cook, stirring, over medium-low heat until heated through. For the high-protein version, place the ground beef and turmeric in a large skillet set over medium heat and cook, stirring continually, until the meat is browned. Drain the grease, add the potato mixture, mix well, and heat through. Serve as is, or as a sandwich in warm pita bread.

Yield: 4 servings

Low-protein version
Calories per serving: 148
Protein: 4 g
Sodium: 41 mg
Potassium: 418 mg (unleached potatoes)
Phosphorus: 79 mg

High-protein version
Calories per serving: 330
Protein: 27 g
Sodium: 89 mg
Potassium: 424 mg (unleached potatoes)
Phosphorus: 182 mg

Pasta Salad

- 2 tablespoons rice-wine or other mild vinegar
- 2 tablespoons canola or other vegetable oil
- ½ cup low-fat mayonnaise
- 2 tablespoons ground Parmesan cheese
- 2 tablespoons chopped fresh basil or 1 tablespoon dried
- 1 tablespoon dried thyme
- 2½ cups cooked rotini or other small pasta
- ⅔ cup lightly cooked green peas, fresh or frozen

High-protein version:

- ¾ pound broiled, roasted, or grilled diced chicken or whole shrimp, and 1 small tomato, seeded and chopped

Low-protein version:

- 1½ cups chopped cooked asparagus or broccoli, or raw green or red bell pepper

Combine the vinegar, oil, mayonnaise, Parmesan, basil, and thyme in a large bowl. Add the pasta and peas, and toss to coat. For the low-protein version, add the additional diced vegetables and toss. For the high-protein version, add the meat and tomato and toss. Serve vegetable pasta salad chilled, the meat pasta salad at room temperature.

Yield: 4 servings

Low-protein version (using ¾ cup each asparagus and red bell pepper)
Calories per serving: 296
Protein: 7 g
Sodium: 183 mg
Potassium: 245 mg
Phosphorus: 98 mg

High-protein version (using chicken)
Calories per serving: 378
Protein: 26 g
Sodium: 237 mg
Potassium: 359 mg
Phosphorus: 246 mg

Sweet Baked Corn

3 eggs
1 cup half-and-half
½ cup nondairy creamer
3 tablespoons honey
2 tablespoons unsalted margarine or butter, melted
3 cups cooked corn kernels, fresh or frozen
Vegetable cooking spray

Preheat the oven to 400°F. In a medium bowl, beat the eggs, half-and-half, creamer, honey, and margarine. Stir in the corn. Pour the mixture into an 8 x 8-inch cake pan coated with spray oil. Set the pan in a larger pan and add enough warm water to reach one quarter of the way up the smaller pan. Bake about 35 minutes, or until brown on top and firm to the touch.

Yield: 6 servings

Calories per serving: 247
Protein: 7 g
Sodium: 62 mg
Potassium: 228 mg
Phosphorus: 133 mg

Saffron Rice

2	tablespoons olive or other vegetable oil
1	clove garlic, minced
1	medium onion, diced
⅛	teaspoon ground saffron
1	cup peas, fresh or frozen
¾	cup rice
1½	cups low-sodium chicken broth or water
1	medium tomato, seeded and diced
3	tablespoons chopped fresh parsley
	Dash Tabasco

Heat the oil in a large skillet set over medium heat. Sauté the garlic and onion until the onion is transluscent. Add the saffron, peas, rice, and broth, and stir well. Bring to a boil, then turn down the heat, cover, and simmer 15 minutes. Stir in the tomato and 2 tablespoons of the parsley, and Tabasco. Cover and cook 5 minutes more, or until all the liquid has been absorbed. Sprinkle with the remaining 1 tablespoon parsley and serve.

Yield: 6 servings

Calories per serving: 152
Protein: 3 g
Sodium: 31 mg
Potassium: 126 mg
Phosphorus: 55 mg

Stewed Apples and Pears

2	medium apples, peeled and sliced
1	medium pear, peeled and sliced
¾	cup water
⅓	cup honey
1	tablespoon cornstarch
¼	cup nondairy creamer
½	teaspoon ground cinnamon
⅛	teaspoon ground nutmeg

Put the apple, pear, water, and honey in a medium saucepan set over medium heat and cook 5 minutes. Stir the cornstarch into the creamer and add it to the fruit mixture. Add the cinnamon and nutmeg, increase the heat to medium-high and cook 3 to 5 minutes, stirring continually. Reduce the heat, cover, and simmer, stirring occasionally, 10 minutes, or until the fruit is tender. Serve warm on its own or with vanilla ice cream.

Yield: 4 servings

Calories per serving: 175
Protein: 0.4 g
Sodium: 9 mg
Potassium: 161 mg
Phosphorus: 19 mg

Dijon Carrots and Zucchini

2	tablespoons vegetable oil or water
2	medium carrots, peeled and cut into 2-inch sticks
2	medium zucchini, cut into 2-inch sticks
1	teaspoon cider vinegar
1	teaspoon honey
1½	teaspoons Dijon mustard

Heat the oil in a medium skillet set over medium heat. Add the carrots, cover, and cook 10 minutes, stirring twice. Add the zucchini and cook 5 more minutes, or until the vegetables are just tender. Mix the vinegar, honey, and mustard in a small bowl, add to the cooked vegetables, and toss to coat. Serve warm.

Yield: 4 servings

Calories per serving: 90
Protein: 1 g
Sodium: 39 mg
Potassium: 241 mg
Phosphorus: 33 mg

Lemony Potatoes

1½	pounds potatoes, peeled and cut into 1-inch cubes
4	tablespoons unsalted butter or margarine
1	tablespoon lemon juice
1	teaspoon grated lemon zest
3	tablespoons chopped fresh parsley
1	tablespoon chopped fresh chives
⅛	teaspoon ground black pepper

Soak the potatoes in water overnight to remove some of the potassium. Boil them in unsalted water about 15 minutes, or until tender. Melt the butter in a small saucepan and add the lemon juice, zest, parsley, chives, and pepper. Put the drained potatoes in a serving bowl, add the hot lemon butter, and toss to coat.

Yield: 6 servings

Calories per serving: 166
Protein: 2 g
Sodium: 7 mg
Potassium: 389 mg (unleached potatoes)
Phosphorus: 48 mg

Stuffed Peppers

4	green bell peppers
3	medium onions, diced
⅓	pound mushrooms, diced
2	cloves garlic, minced
1	tablespoon water
¼	teaspoon dried oregano
¼	teaspoon dried basil
⅛	teaspoon ground black pepper
1	cup cooked white rice
2	tablespoons grated Parmesan cheese
3	tablespoons low-sodium tomato paste
⅓	cup low-fat cottage cheese
	Vegetable cooking spray

Preheat the oven to 350°F. Dice one of the green peppers. Put the onions, mushrooms, garlic, and diced pepper in a large skillet set over medium heat. Add the water and cook 5 to 7 minutes, or until the onion is transluscent. Stir in the oregano, basil, black pepper, rice, Parmesan, tomato paste, and cottage cheese. Cut the remaining 3 green peppers in half, remove the seeds, and stuff them with the vegetable-and-cheese mixture. Place them in a baking dish coated with spray oil and bake 1 hour, or until the peppers are soft.

Yield: 6 servings

Calories per serving: 112
Protein: 5 g
Sodium: 99 mg
Potassium: 376 mg
Phosphorus: 111 mg

Baked Onions

2 medium mild-flavored onions
2 teaspoons unsalted butter or margarine
4 teaspoons sherry
¼ teaspoon dried thyme

Preheat the oven to 325°F. Peel the onions and cut out the core. Wrap each onion in a double thickness of foil, leaving the opening on top exposed. Fill the cavity of each onion with half the butter, sherry, and thyme. Place them on a baking sheet and cook 30 to 45 minutes, or until very tender.

Yield: 2 servings

Calories per serving: 83
Protein: 1 g
Sodium: 4 mg
Potassium: 184 mg
Phosphorus: 39 mg

Buttery Cabbage

4	teaspoons unsalted butter or margarine
1	small head green cabbage, cut into large bite-sized pieces
4	tablespoons white vinegar
½	teaspoon ground black pepper

Melt the butter in a large skillet set over medium heat. Add the cabbage, vinegar, and pepper and cook, stirring occasionally, about 7 minutes, or until the cabbage is partly transluscent and tender. Serve warm with vinegar and pepper on the side.

Yield: 4 servings

Calories per serving: 106
Protein: 3 g
Sodium: 26 mg
Potassium: 326 mg
Phosphorus: 50 mg

Rice and Spinach Casserole

1½	cups rice
	10-ounce package frozen spinach
3	tablespoons grated Parmesan cheese
2	tablespoons chopped fresh parsley
1	teaspoon dried oregano
1	teaspoon dried thyme
⅛	teaspoon ground black pepper
2	eggs
1	cup low-fat milk
	Vegetable cooking spray

Preheat the oven to 350°F. Prepare the rice and the spinach according to package instructions, omitting any added salt. Squeeze the cooked spinach to remove as much water as possible. In a large bowl, mix the rice, spinach, Parmesan, parsley, oregano, thyme, and pepper. Beat the eggs and milk in a small bowl and add it to the rice-and-spinach mixture. Mix well and transfer to a large casserole dish coated with spray oil. Bake about 30 minutes, or until bubbly around the edges. Sprinkle with Parmesan and serve warm.

Yield: 5 servings

Calories per serving: 166
Protein: 9 g
Sodium: 170 mg
Potassium: 311 mg
Phosphorus: 169 mg

Sweet-and-Sour Orangy Beets

- 4 medium beets
- 3 tablespoons water
- 3 tablespoons white vinegar
- 3 tablespoons packed brown sugar
- 2 tablespoons grated orange zest
- 2 teaspoons cornstarch
- ⅛ teaspoon ground clove

Cook the beets in boiling water about 25 minutes, or until tender, or microwave with a little water, loosely covered, at full power about 2 minutes. Slip off the skins, cut the beets into quarters, and set aside. Put the water, vinegar, sugar, zest, cornstarch, and clove in a medium saucepan set over medium-high heat and cook 2 minutes, stirring continually. Add the beets, reduce the heat to medium, and cook 5 minutes. Serve warm.

Yield: 4 servings

Calories per serving: 103
Protein: 1 g
Sodium: 65 mg
Potassium: 292 mg
Phosphorus: 36 mg

Blueberry-Yogurt Cake

	Vegetable cooking spray
2	cups flour
1	cup sugar
½	teaspoon baking soda
1	tablespoon baking powder
1	teaspoon ground nutmeg
⅔	cup unsweetened applesauce
2	eggs
1	cup low-fat vanilla yogurt
2	cups blueberries, fresh or thawed frozen unsweetened

Preheat the oven to 350°F. and coat a 9 x 9-inch baking pan with spray oil. In a large bowl, combine the flour, sugar, baking soda, baking powder, and nutmeg. In a small bowl, combine the applesauce, eggs, and yogurt. Add the wet to the dry ingredients and mix until just combined. Gently fold in the blueberries (do not over-mix). Pour the batter into the prepared pan and bake 50 minutes, or until brown at the edges.

Yield: 16 servings

Calories per serving: 143
Protein: 3 g
Sodium: 114 mg
Potassium: 77 mg
Phosphorus: 140 mg

Rice Pudding with Sweet Cherries

½   cup rice
1   cup low-fat milk
1   cup nondairy creamer
½   cup dried or frozen sweet cherries (without phosphorus-containing preservatives)
2   eggs
¼   cup honey
1   teaspoon vanilla extract
     Pinch nutmeg

Put the rice, milk, creamer, and cherries in the top of a double boiler. Cover and cook 45 minutes over low heat. In a large bowl, beat the eggs and honey. Add the rice mixture in small amounts to the egg mixture, blending well after each addition. Return the pudding to the double boiler and cook, stirring continually, about 3 minutes, or until it thickens. Remove from the heat and stir in the vanilla and nutmeg. Serve warm or chilled.

Yield: 6 servings

Calories per serving: 232
Protein: 5 g
Sodium: 62 mg
Potassium: 211 mg
Phosphorus: 118 mg

Apple Cake

Vegetable cooking spray
2 eggs
1 teaspoon vanilla extract
1 cup sugar
4 medium apples, peeled and diced
1 cup flour
2 teaspoons cinnamon
2 teaspoons baking powder

Preheat the oven to 350°F. and coat a 9 x 9-inch baking pan with spray oil. In a large bowl, mix the eggs, vanilla, and sugar. Fold in the apple. In a small bowl, mix the flour, cinnamon, and baking powder. Add this to the wet ingredients and mix just to combine. Pour the batter into the prepared pan and bake 15 to 20 minutes, or until brown around the edges.

Yield: 16 servings

Calories per serving: 108
Protein: 2 g
Sodium: 55 mg
Potassium: 54 mg
Phosphorus: 81 mg

Shortbread Cookies

Cornstarch, which is very low in protein, is substituted for some flour in this recipe.

1½	cups flour plus more for dusting
1⅓	cups cornstarch
¾	cup sugar
½	pound (2 sticks) unsalted margarine
1	egg yolk
2	tablespoons cream or milk
2	teaspoons vanilla extract
2	teaspoons grated lemon zest
	Vegetable cooking spray

Put the flour, cornstarch, and sugar in a large bowl and mix to combine. Cut the margarine into the flour mixture using a pastry blender. Mix the egg yolk, cream, vanilla, and zest in a small bowl. Add this to the dry ingredients, blending with a fork until the mixture forms a dough. Knead lightly until the dough becomes smooth. Cover with plastic wrap and refrigerate at least 1 hour and up to 24 hours. Preheat the oven to 400°F. and lightly coat a cookie sheet with spray oil. Form the dough into walnut-size balls and place them 2 inches apart on the prepared cookie sheet. Press each ball flat with a floured fork. Bake 15 minutes, or until golden.

Variations:
Chocolate Shortbread Cookies: Omit the lemon zest and add 2 tablespoons cocoa.
Cinnamon Shortbread Cookies: Omit the lemon zest and vanilla and add 2 teaspoons ground cinnamon.

Shortbread Cookies with Jam: Before baking, make an indention in each cookie and fill it with a little jam.

Yield: 25 2-cookie servings

Calories per serving: 148
Protein: 1 g
Sodium: 2 mg
Potassium: 13 mg
Phosphorus: 14 mg

Lemon Pie

- ⅓ cup lemon juice
- 2 teaspoons grated lemon zest
- 4 tablespoons unsalted butter or margarine, melted
- ¼ cup low-fat milk
- 1¾ cups sugar
- 2 tablespoons flour
- 4 eggs, lightly beaten
- 9-inch unbaked pie crust

Preheat the oven to 350°F. Add the lemon juice and zest to the melted butter. Allow to cool slightly and stir in the milk. Mix the sugar, flour, and eggs in a medium bowl and stir in the butter mixture. Pour the filling into the crust and bake about 50 minutes, or until browned on top. Allow the pie to come to room temperature before serving.

Yield: 10 servings

Calories per serving: 352
Protein: 4 g
Sodium: 128 mg
Potassium: 63 mg
Phosphorus: 59 mg

Peach Crisp

Vegetable cooking spray
¾ cup sugar
5 tablespoons unsalted butter or margarine
½ cup flour
⅓ cup rolled oats
½ teaspoon ground nutmeg
4 cups fresh or frozen unsweetened peach slices, or other fresh or frozen unsweetened fruit

Preheat the oven to 325°F. and coat an 8 x 8-inch casserole dish with spray oil. Cream the sugar and butter. Combine the flour, oats, and nutmeg, and add it to the butter mixture; the topping mixture will be crumbly. Arrange the fruit in the casserole dish and distribute the topping over it. Bake 30 to 35 minutes, or until bubbling at the edges and brown on top.

Variation, using canned, sweetened fruit: Omit the sugar and increase the flour to ¾ cup and the rolled oats to ½ cup.

Yield: 8 servings

Calories per serving: 219
Protein: 2 g
Sodium: 1 mg
Potassium: 191 mg
Phosphorus: 37 mg

Appendix A:
Seasoning with Herbs and Spices (Abridged)

Fran Rukenbrod, M.Ed., R.D., L.D.N.

On a low-fat, low-sodium diet? Do your meals seem bland-tasting? Try using herbs and spices to enhance the flavor of foods.

Today, packaged herbs are available nearly everywhere, and in some stores you can purchase dry herbs by the ounce. Fresh herbs are even better. If you are able to obtain fresh herbs for only a few months of the year, you may want to consider drying your own or freezing them.

The most common way to dry herbs is to tie them in a bunch and hang them out of the sun, in a room with even heat. When dried, they can be stored in a tightly sealed container.

To freeze fresh herbs, chop them and place them in ice cube trays, adding water and freezing. Remove the cubes and seal them in labeled freezer bags. One tablespoon of fresh herbs equals ½ to 1 teaspoon of dried herbs.

Other Storage Tips

- Keep herbs and spices in tightly closed containers away from the heat of the stove. Consider replacing them if they are more than a year old.
- Paprika and cayenne pepper are susceptible to insect invasion, so consider storing them in the refrigerator.
- Fresh herbs keep longer when stored with cut ends in water and the tops lightly covered with a plastic bag.
- Fresh ginger may be kept in the freezer. Place whole root in a sealed bag in the freezer. Frozen ginger is easy to peel and grate and lasts well.

The use of flavorings is a very individual matter. As a creative cook, you really don't need any guidelines, but for those of you who need a little help, here are a few generally accepted suggestions about what herb goes well with what food.

Allspice. Dried spice berries. Allspice tastes of cinnamon, cloves, and nutmeg—hence the name. Excellent in spice cakes and cookies; plum, peach, and apple pies; breads; steamed puddings; and barbecue sauce, ketchup, and pickles.

Basil. Herb with sweet clovelike taste. Varieties include sweet basil, small-leaved bush basil, dark opal, and lemon basil. Essential herb for Italian food, especially with eggs, tomatoes, pasta, chicken, fish, and shellfish.

Bay Leaf. Pungent, woodsy herb with sturdy leaves and faint cinnamon taste. Good with meat and/or bean stews, game, pot roasts; adds unusual note to rice pudding and custards.

Cayenne. Red pepper of the capsicum family most often used dried. Best used in any dish for a little heat. Add cayenne by the pinch.

Chili Powder. Commercial mix of ground chile peppers, cumin, oregano, and other herbs and spices. Use in bean and meat stews and soups; with eggs, egg substitutes, and cheese.

Chives. Delicate herb with light onion or garlic taste. Decorative as well as useful garden herb. Excellent in soups with fish and shellfish, eggs and egg substitutes.

Clove. Spice of winter holidays, pungent and sweet. A few whole cloves stuck in an onion flavor stocks, but most are added ground to spice cakes and cookies, quick breads and fruit pies. Use judiciously with sweet potatoes, winter squash, and carrots.

Coriander/Cilantro. Nutty-tasting seeds are called coriander. Cilantro is the herb. Use whole seeds for pickles and ground for baking. Cilantro is an essential herb for Mexican, Latin American, and Asian cooking. Use with rice, fish, shellfish, poultry, vegetables, salsas, and salads. Add the fresh herb at the last minute before serving.

Cumin. Small, hot, bitter seed. Essential spice for curry and chili powder mixtures. Good with curried vegetables, fish, lamb, and poultry as well as with cheese, chutney, and yogurt dip.

Dill. Seeds have delicate caraway taste. Seeds are the more pungent. Both seeds and herb are used for pickles. Use seeds with rice and fish dishes and fresh dill leaves with eggs, egg substitutes, cheeses, yogurt, seafood, chicken, cucumbers, green beans, potatoes, tomatoes, and beets.

Fennel Seeds. Slight licorice flavor, similar to anise. Favorite for Scandinavian breads, cakes, and cookies. Also good with fish soup, and with vegetables, in salads and salad dressing.

Garlic. Strong or mild flavor depending on use. Has nutty, sweet taste when used alone. Heads or bulbs should be large, firm, and tight skinned. Use in tomato dishes, soups, dips, sauces, salads, salad dressings, dill pickles, meat, poultry, fish, stews, marinades, and breads.

Ginger. Versatile spice with bite and aroma. Important to dozens of cuisines, from Jamaican to German to Chinese. Use ground dried judiciously in cakes, cookies, fruit and squash pies, custard, rice, and marinades. Use crystallized and preserved in cakes and cookies. Use fresh sliced or grated in marinades and with fish, poultry, pork, and vegetables.

Marjoram. Herb that is first cousin to oregano with similar but more delicate taste. Use in almost any fish, meat, poultry, egg, or vegetable dish, and in tomato sauce.

Mint. Herb with refreshing scent and cool taste. Of more than 30 varieties, peppermint and spearmint are best known. Lemon, orange, and apple mint have distinct fruit taste. Best used in Middle Eastern yogurt and grain dishes (tabbouleh), salads; with peas, beans, corn, and potatoes; in jellies, fruit salads, desserts, and iced tea.

Nutmeg. Sweet, nutty spice seed of the nutmeg tree, the size of an olive. Best in soups, with vegetables—beans, broccoli, carrots, cauliflower, spinach, Brussels sprouts, onions—but especially for cakes, cookies, pies, pastries, and custard.

Oregano. Herb with pungent marjoram taste. Use with fish, meat, poultry, dried beans, cheese, eggs; in vegetable soup; with tomatoes, mushrooms, peppers, summer squash, and eggplant. Essential herb for Italian, Greek, and Mexican cooking.

Paprika. Ground spice of dried capsicum peppers. Good in cooked salads—especially potato and egg—salad dressing, dips; with fish, shellfish, and poultry. Essential for goulash and paprikash.

Parsley. Crisp herb with celery flavor. Of two common varieties—Italian flat leaf and curly leaf—flat leaf has the stronger flavor. Use curly parsley for garnishing. Excellent in soups, stocks and tomato sauces, salads and salad dressings; with poultry, game, meats, fish and shellfish, dried beans, and vegetables—from artichokes to zucchini.

Rosemary. Needlelike leaves with strong piny scent and flavor. Best with game, poultry, and meats, especially grilled. Add judiciously to mushrooms, roasted potatoes, stuffing, and olive oil breads.

Sage. Herb with musky flavor. Silver-green leaves make sage a decorative garden plant. Excellent and best known for poultry and stuffing. Use judiciously with chicken, pork, cheese, eggplant, and dried bean stews and soups.

Tarragon. Herb with mild licorice flavor. Best with chicken, veal, fish, shellfish, eggs; in mayonnaise and salad dressing; with tomatoes, mushrooms, and carrots.

Thyme. Herb with tiny leaves and minty, tea-like flavor. Many varieties include lemon, orange, English, and French thyme. Essential herb for fish and clam chowder, and stuffing. Excellent with fish and shellfish, poultry, tomatoes, beans, eggplant, mushrooms, potatoes, and summer squash.

Turmeric. Brilliant yellow ground spice. Essential to mustard, curry powder, pickles, and relishes; also used in moderation for its yellow color in rice dishes.

Appendix B

A Blank Food Record Worksheet					
	Number of choices				
Food Items	Starch	Veget.	Fruit	Meat (1 oz)	Dairy
Goal					
TOTAL					

Date: _____

		Amount		
Fat (1 t)	Extra calories	Protein (g)	High-quality?	Sodium (mg)

Resources

Organizations

American Association of Kidney Patients
100 South Ashley Drive, Suite 280
Tampa, FL 33602
(813) 223-7099; (800) 749-2257
Publishes a magazine called Renalife.

American Dietetic Association
216 West Jackson Boulevard
Chicago, IL 60606-6995
(312) 899-0040

Contemporary Dialysis, Inc.
6300 Variel Avenue, Suite I
Woodland Hills, CA 91367
(818) 704-5555
Publishes a magazine called For Patients Only.

National Kidney and Urologic Diseases Information
Clearinghouse
Box NKUDIC, 9000 Rockville Pike
Bethesda, MD 20892
(301) 654-4415

National Kidney Foundation
30 East Thirty-third Street
New York, NY 10016
(212) 889-2210; (800) 622-9010
Publishes a magazine called The Kidney *and a wide
range of pamphlets and other literature on a variety of
topics.*

Specialty Products

Diamond Crystal Specialty Foods for Modified Diets
P.O. Box 224
Amherst, NY 14226
(800) 827-6763
Call for a free catalog.

Med-Diet Laboratories, Inc.
3050 Ranchview Lane
Plymouth, MN 55447
(800) 633-3438
Call for a free catalog.

Further Reading

Diet and Lifestyle

T. P. Ahlstrom, *Kidney Patient's Book: New Treatment, New Hope,* 1991, Great Issues Press, P.O. Box 1336, Delran, NJ 08075. *Discusses a more conservative treatment than what we recommend.*

E. T. Oberley and T. D. Oberley, *Understanding Your New Life with Dialysis,* 1992, Charles C. Thomas, Publisher, 2600 South First Street, Springfield, IL 62794-9265. (217) 789-8980.

R. H. Phillips, *Coping with Kidney Failure,* 1987, Avery Publishing Group, Garden City Park, NY.

Protein Wise for Self-Monitoring, Nutrition Section, Graduate School of Public Health, University of Pittsburgh, 130 DeSoto Street, Room 503, Pittsburgh, PA 15213. (412) 624-3203.

D. Reader and M. Franz, *Pass the Pepper Please!,* 1988, Diabetes Center, Inc., P.O. Box 739, Wayzata, MN 55391.

Cookbooks

American Heart Association, *Cooking Without Your Salt Shaker,* 1991, National Center, 7320 Greenville Avenue, Dallas, TX 75431.

Amgen, Inc., Dept. of Professional Services, *Living Well on Dialysis: A Cookbook for Patients and Their Families,* 1840 DeHavilland Drive, Thousand Oaks, CA 91320-1789. (800) 772-6436. *Single copy free.*

E. Levy Klein, *Skinny Spices: 50 Nifty Homemade Spice Blends That Can Make Any Diet Delicious,* 1990, Surrey Books, Chicago, IL.

Low Protein Cookery: Recipes, Helpful Hints and Information Relating to Protein-Restricted Diets, 1992, University of Alberta Hospitals, Nutrition and Food Services, 8440-112 Street, Edmonton, Alberta T6G 2B7 Canada. (403) 492-6882.

M. Peters, *Renal Gourmet, Or What to Cook When Your Kidneys Quit: A Cook Book by a Kidney Patient,* 1991, Emenar, Inc., 1545 Lee Street, Suite 6100, Des Plaines, IL 60018. (708) 299-1226.

V. E. Schuett, *Low Protein Cookery for PKU,* University of Wisconsin Press, 114 North Murray St., Madison, WI 53715. *PKU is another medical condition that requires protein restriction.*

M. Vennegoor, ed., *Enjoying Food on a Renal Diet,* 1992, Ultrapharm Limited, P.O. Box 18, Henley on Thames, Oxfordshire, RG9 2AW England.

Index

Italic entries refer to recipes.